LOSE WEIGHT
GET HEALTHY
& BE HAPPY

The Rice Diet is the Right Diet, for you!

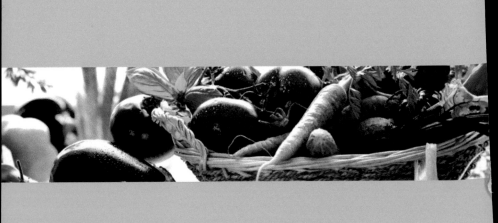

LOSE WEIGHT GET HEALTHY & BE HAPPY

The Rice Diet is the Right Diet, for you!

Douglas Jay Sprung, MD, FACG, FACP
and Denise Sprung, MSW

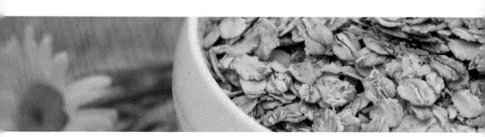

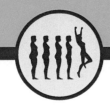

Visit us on the Web! www.RiceDietCF.com

Book Design by Brian Margolis, Crank Communications

First Edition

For more information:
info@ricedietcf.com | 407-261-0000 | *www.RiceDietCF.com*

Printed in the USA

This book is dedicated to the memory of Dr. Walter Kempner, the originator of the Rice Diet; to the thousands of people whose lives have been transformed by the Diet; and especially to you, for being motivated to lose weight for a healthier, higher-quality and happier life.

IMPORTANT

Do not begin this diet without a doctor's supervision if you have any medical problems and are taking medications for those problems.

If you are taking medication for high blood pressure, diabetes, arthritis or heart disease, or are taking blood thinners such as Coumadin or Warfarin, do not begin this diet until you get medical clearance from your doctor. Once you have received medical consent and approval, your doctor must continue to monitor you and your progress throughout the course of your diet.

INTRODUCTION
THE RICE DIET IS THE RIGHT DIET

ONCE UPON A TIME there was a woman who desperately wanted to lose weight, but she didn't want to do the work required to lose the pounds. Instead, she wanted to lose weight magically. Then one day, the Weight Loss Fairy appeared before the woman, waved her magic wand—and behold! The woman instantly lost all her excess pounds and lived happily ever after!

Ah, if only there was a Weight Loss Fairy who could make the pounds disappear with a wave of her magic wand. Then everyone would be trim and healthy—and we wouldn't have written this book! But like all good things in life, weight loss doesn't happen magically. Instead, it happens when motivated people adopt a sensible, doable weight loss plan—and stick to it. The Rice Diet is the sensible, doable weight loss regimen that will help you lose weight, and this book will serve to show you how.

The Rice Diet was developed in 1940 at Duke University by Dr. Walter Kempner, a bright, compassionate physician who preached the benefits of obesity prevention long before it became a national health issue. As

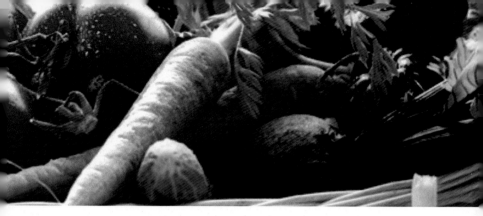

the name implies, rice is a staple of the Diet. At the beginning, you'll go through a short period of eating rice and fruits, to adjust your body to your new and healthier food intake.

Your diet will then expand to eating vegetables, poultry, fish and lean meats, and ultimately, pasta, low-sodium breads, crackers and more. The Rice Diet is a normal, balanced, satisfying and filling diet.

Over the years, the Diet has helped thousands of people lose weight and, just as important, keep the weight off. We first learned about the Diet when Dr. Sprung was a student at Duke University School of Medicine. He was impressed by how the Rice Diet worked. REALLY impressed. But there was a catch: the program was only available on the Duke campus, meaning you had to go there, enroll in the program and stay for several weeks or months. Not exactly convenient! Now, with a few modifications to the program—and the writing of this book—the benefits of the Rice Diet are available to anyone, anywhere.

This book provides the blueprint for building a trimmer, healthier, happier you. While it calls for changes in your diet and what you eat, they are beneficial changes. You'll enjoy a wide variety of tasty foods and meals on the Rice Diet, rest assured. Exercise is also a cornerstone of the diet, but we're talking about the kind of physical activity most anyone can do. Once you get settled into your diet regimen, you'll appreciate healthful eating and beneficial exercise—and of course, losing all those pounds and gaining a happier, more satisfying life than you've ever imagined.

What does it take to succeed on the Rice Diet? That's simple. It takes you. First, you need to be motivated to lose weight and keep it off. You must also be willing to change the habits and behaviors that led to you being overweight. And you must commit to staying with the Diet, and making it a central part of your (healthier, happier) life. Admittedly, doing these things is not always easy. But neither is it impossible. Hardly! The fact is, thousands and thousands of people just like you have lost thousands and thousands of pounds with the Rice Diet. All they did was stick with the program—and the program stuck with them. You can do it, too.

As we end these opening remarks, we want you to visualize the end results of your Rice Diet experience. Imagine the simple joy of being lighter, trimmer, healthier and more energetic. Imagine how good that feels, physically and mentally! Imagine decreasing or eliminating the medicines you take, and even reversing your medical conditions—this too can happen with the Rice Diet. Think of the new clothes you can wear, and all the compliments you'll get from family and friends. Accept

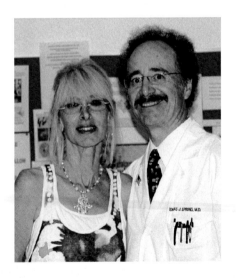

them with pride: You deserve them—because you've earned them. Finally, imagine all the new and wonderful possibilities for your life when you replace your "live-to-eat" mindset with an "eat-to-live" one. You'll have a new image of yourself, a new outlook on life, and a renewed sense of enthusiasm for waking up and taking on the day.

Does all this sound good to you? GREAT. Now let's get started!

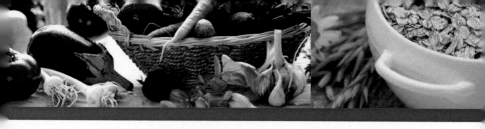

For your convenience and easy reference, we divided this book into two parts:

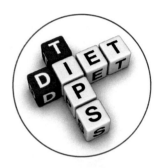

Part One, The Rice Diet Lifestyle
Discusses the practices and habits (along with tips) that are essential to your dieting success.

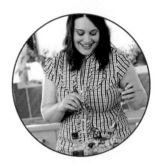

Part Two, The Tools for Success
Includes weekly menus and recipes, a sample Rice Diet Journal, and other useful information pertaining to your diet. Read and reread this book often as a guide to, and inspiration for, living the Ricer Life!

Additional resources are available to you in the appendix of this book.

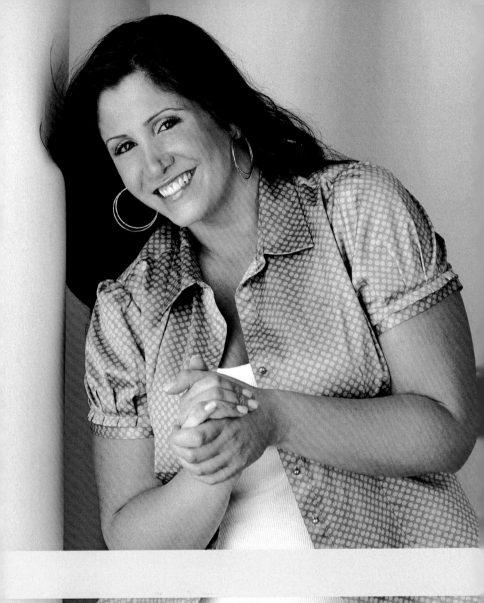

PART ONE
THE RICE DIET LIFESTYLE

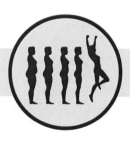

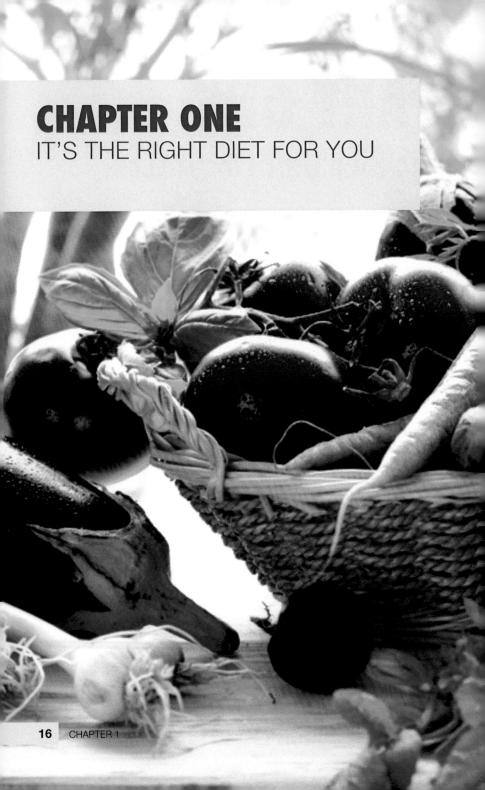

CHAPTER ONE
IT'S THE RIGHT DIET FOR YOU

"Don't talk about dieting...do it."
- Dr. Walter Kempner

CONGRATULATIONS on your commitment to improve your health and your life through the Rice Diet. **You are now a Ricer,** one of thousands of people who have transformed their lives through this sensible, proven-effective diet. You have made an excellent choice, and if you stick with the program, you'll be rewarded with a new, healthier, happier you. In this chapter, we'll explain what the Rice Diet is, how it works, and what it takes to make it work for you.

LET'S START WITH A BRIEF DESCRIPTION

The Rice Diet is designed to help people who suffer from obesity and related conditions, such as heart disease, high cholesterol, arthritis, diabetes and hypertension. The diet features a variety of popular foods including fruits, grains, fish, poultry, lean meats, vegetables and more. These foods are nutritious, filling and satisfying while low in calories. The Rice Diet also emphasizes regular exercise as a way to regulate caloric intake and burn off calories. The diet should initially be under medical supervision to assure that it is compatible with the individual's medical conditions and needs.

The Rice Diet is one of the few diets that has shown documented medical evidence of success in treating a myriad of health problems.

Emphasizing healthy eating, exercise and a positive mental attitude, the Rice Diet is a "good for life" diet that can be followed throughout life to maximize the individual's health and happiness. Truly, it is not just a diet, but a healthy lifestyle regimen.

We'll go into greater detail throughout this book, but that's a good start.

WHAT'S SO SPECIAL ABOUT THE RICE DIET?

That's a good question, especially if you've tried other diets without success. You want a diet that works for you, and there are a number of reasons why the Rice Diet is the one. But remember, there is no one waving a magic wand to enable you to lose the weight. The Rice Diet works, if you're willing to do the work to gain success!

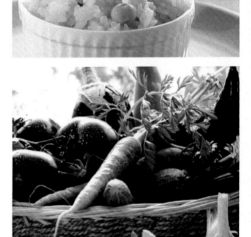

For starters, the Rice Diet consists of typical, everyday foods, many of which you're probably already eating. That makes it fairly easy to get started on and stay with. The meals and snacks you'll enjoy are tasty, filling and satisfying, and there's a wide variety to choose from. You won't grow bored with your food selections and you won't feel deprived in quality or quantity. At the same time, the diet is free of excessive fats, sugar, cholesterol and added salt, which are the big culprits in obesity and a host of other serious medical problems. On the Rice Diet, you can eat delicious, healthy foods while avoiding all the unhealthy choices that contributed to your weight problem and health issues.

Exercise is another feature of the Rice Diet—and another reason why it's the Right Diet for You. If you're presently "exercise-challenged," don't worry. Before they get with the program, most Ricers are! As you'll see though, the exercise required by the diet is both doable and enjoyable. Exercise of course helps burn off calories, but that's not the only benefit. Regular exercise can also help lower the risk of just about every medical nightmare you want to avoid—cancer, diabetes, heart disease, stroke, depression, osteoporosis, you name it. Regular exercise gives you more energy, helps you sleep better, helps you handle stress better and improves your self-esteem. Imagine all these benefits—and they're yours free with the Rice Diet (okay, you may have to spring for a pair of walking shoes, but you get the point).

Baseball Hall of Famer Yogi Berra once said, "Baseball is 90% mental, the other half is physical." Without commenting on Mr. Berra's math skills, let's just say that like baseball, dieting has a mental as well as a physical component. Dieting isn't just about what you eat; it's also about how you think about food, how you feel about yourself and your life, and a host of other issues. If you don't address the thinking processes that contribute to your obesity, you'll never shed weight. Fortunately, the Rice Diet gives you the tools to think healthy as well as eat healthy. Through journaling, positive attitude exercises, lifestyle changes, activity recommendations and other techniques, the Diet can help you look like a new person on the outside by making you a happier person on the inside.

YOU KNOW YOU HAVE AN EATING PROBLEM WHEN...
1. You eat to deal with stress and worry
2. Eating makes you feel loved and cared for
3. You eat to reward yourself
4. Eating makes you feel less lonely
5. Eating allows you to avoid intimacy
6. Eating as much as you want makes you feel powerful
7. Eating helps control your anger or sadness
8. Eating gives you something to look forward to

In a nutshell, the Rice Diet isn't just a diet. It's much more than that, and intentionally so—because the Rice Diet is one of the few that addresses all the issues that cause your obesity. And that may be the greatest beauty of the diet. It's actually a lifestyle: a great, wonderful, liberating lifestyle that transforms and improves your life not just at mealtime, but all the time!

THE 10 COMMANDMENTS (OF THE RICE DIET)

1. Thou Shalt Be Motivated—Motivation is key to the Rice Diet, and we'll go into this in greater detail later. For right now, it's enough to know that this is the First Commandment—and with good reason. Motivation is the key to success in most every phase of life, including weight loss.

2. Thou Shalt Exercise Daily—If you're thinking "No way can I do that!" let us tell you something: you can! In fact, we'll bet you dollars to doughnuts (wait, forget about the doughnuts!) you'll soon come to love your daily exercise routine. We'll talk more about exercise in a while.

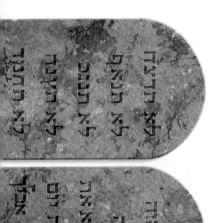

3. Thou Shalt Not Eat In Excess—Portion size and control is very important for losing weight, and it's surprisingly easy when you know how. With the Rice Diet, you'll have that knowledge!

4. Thou Shalt Not Hang Out With People Who Are Not Respectful Of Your Dieting—Surrounding yourself with supportive people is a great aid to your diet program. Don't let the naysayers or the "one triple fudge sundae won't hurt you" crowd keep you from achieving your dream of health and happiness!

5. Thou Shalt Adhere To Your Diet Until You Attain Your Ideal Weight—This is the Holy Grail. Commit to it, seek it, achieve it.

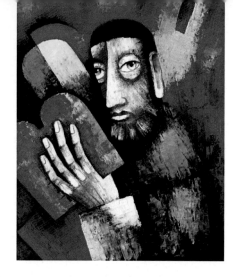

6. Thou Shalt Not Cheat—No one is perfect. We all slip up sometimes, eating something we shouldn't or maybe skipping a day's exercise. But still, that's cheating—and you're only cheating yourself. Resolve to adhere to the program, and if you slip up, be honest with yourself and your physician—then get right back with the program. Later on, we'll discuss slip-ups and how to avoid them.

7. Thou Shalt Reverse Hypertension, Heart Disease, Diabetes and Renal Disease If You Suffer From Them—These are your enemies. The Rice Diet will arm you with the weapons you need to defeat them. Their days are numbered!

8. Thou Shalt Reduce Stress—Stress is a big trigger for overeating and other unhealthy behaviors, and it's important to reduce stress in your life. We'll discuss how a little further in this book.

9. Thou Shalt Prevent New Illnesses By Adhering To The Doctrines Of The Rice Diet—Following the Rice Diet for a lifetime can reduce the chances of getting new illnesses, another reason to commit to the program.

10. Thou Shalt Maintain The Program—It will always work for you if you always work with it.

LOSING WEIGHT: GOOD FOR YOU

The National Institute of Health declares that obesity has risen to epidemic levels in the U.S., with nearly 68% of all adults either overweight or obese. There has also been a recent, alarming rise in childhood obesity. According to one 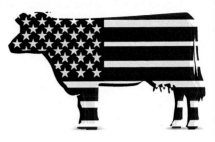 recent study, the economic costs of obesity in the U.S. reach $215 billion annually. Losing weight may not be our patriotic duty, but it sure would make our nation healthier. That's something every American should take an interest in.

MORE QUESTIONS, MORE ANSWERS

Here are some of the basic questions asked about the Rice Diet. If you have additional questions not found here, talk with your physician or visit our Web site at *ricedietcf.com*.

Q: Why is it called the Rice Diet?
Rice is an excellent, low-sodium food. It provides excellent weight loss results when eaten in combination with other approved foods in appropriate portions as part of a controlled diet. Again, the Rice Diet DOES NOT consist of eating rice exclusively. Rather, it features a wide range of popular, everyday foods eaten in combination with rice. You can eat white rice, brown rice, Basmati rice, Jasmine rice, converted rice, Arborio rice, Parboiled rice, whichever type you prefer.

Q: Who can benefit most from the Rice Diet?
The Rice Diet is ideal and proven effective for anyone suffering from obesity or any of the following illnesses:
• Hypertension
• Diabetes

- Coronary artery disease
- Peripheral artery disease
- Strokes, heart attack or heart failure
- Arthritis
- Sleep apnea
- Fatty liver
- Gastro esophageal reflux
- High lipid levels

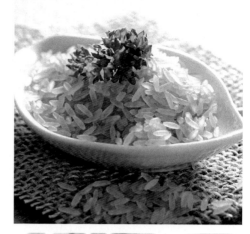

Q: Is this a low-sodium diet?
Absolutely. Most obese people have excess salt in their bodies. Salt attracts water, and in obese people, this results in excess body fluids. Excess salt in the body can contribute to a number of serious medical problems such as hypertension, heart attacks, strokes and heart failure.

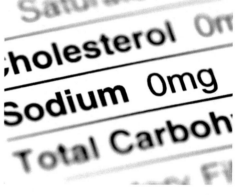

Lowering sodium intake is vitally important for most obese people, and the Rice Diet helps achieve this.

Q: You said the Rice Diet is more than just a diet? What do you mean?
The Rice Diet isn't just a way of eating. It's a lifestyle, a way of living. The Rice Diet incorporates diet, exercise and a positive mental attitude to address all the issues of obesity. Gaining control of your eating habits will also give you more control and confidence in other areas of your life. Taking this holistic approach is one reason why the diet is so successful.

Q: Is this a short-term or a long-term diet?
Successfully managing weight, especially for an obese person, is a

life-long project. Even if you reach your ideal weight in a relatively short period of time, maintaining it, along with all the health benefits, requires long-term commitment. Fortunately, the Rice Diet is designed for the long term. You can begin it today, and enjoy and benefit from it the rest of your life.

Q: What kind of medical supervision does the diet require?
Medical supervision under the Rice Diet varies from person to person. You should consult your doctor and get a routine physical exam including blood work prior to starting the diet, and once you begin, you should meet regularly with your doctor to monitor your progress. **See the Disclaimer at the beginning of this book.**

Q: I've failed with other diets. How can I be SURE I'll succeed with this one?
That's really up to you, because you are the key to success. There's no question that dieting isn't easy, especially for people for whom food has become an obsession or an addiction. Successful dieting requires permanent changes not just in eating habits, but in one's lifestyle. It takes commitment, dedication, effort and a positive attitude. That said, if you really, truly want to succeed with the Rice Diet—you can. There is nothing difficult about the diet itself. You can buy the foods at any grocery store and can cook them easily. The challenging part is committing to your diet and staying with it.

To be successful on the Rice Diet, it's essential to maintain an "I Can" attitude. Since Dr. Kempner introduced it some 70 years ago, thousands and thousands of people have lost weight, rid themselves of obesity, prevented or reversed serious medical conditions and attained new health and happiness by following the Rice Diet. So can you.

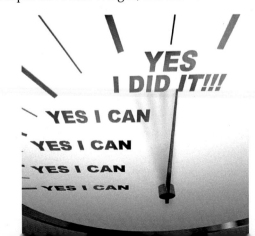

AVOID THE "SEE FOOD" DIET!

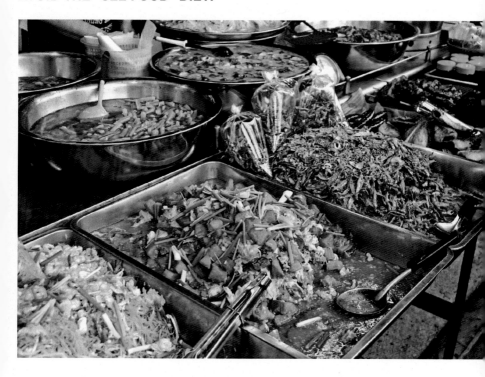

MAKING THE RIGHT CHOICE

When you get right down to it, life is about choices. In just about any situation you come across, you have a choice. You can remain obese, unhealthy, unsatisfied, unfulfilled and unhappy. But if you do, it's because you have chosen so. On the other hand, you can lose weight, regain your health, improve your confidence and self-esteem and enjoy life more than perhaps you ever have. And again, it will be because you have chosen to do so.

The very fact that you are reading this book says loud and clear that you are making the right choice!

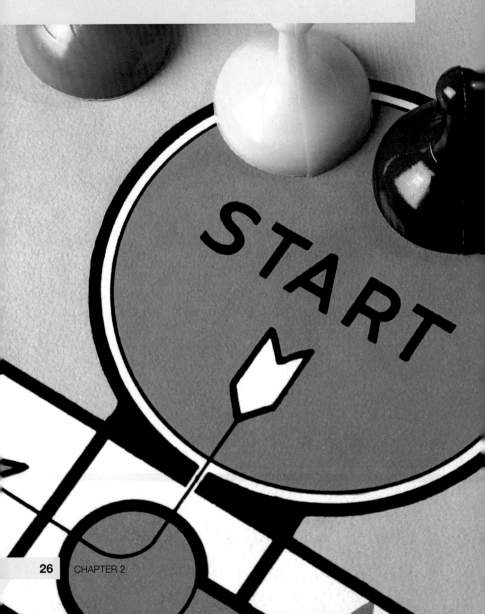

CHAPTER TWO
GETTING STARTED

> ## *"A journey of a thousand miles begins with a single step."*
> ### - Lao Tzu

THE RICE DIET IS A JOURNEY that can take you from obesity to health and happiness, from an unsatisfying life to a quality life. Getting started on your journey requires only a few cooking and measuring items and utensils, a comfortable exercise outfit and some walking shoes, and an introduction to some simple cooking recommendations. Also—and this is very important—before starting your diet: Consult your physician and get a complete physical exam, including the following blood work: CBC, Urine Sodium, CMP, Lipid panel, and TSH.

Now... let's take our first steps.

MEASURING AND COOKING DEVICES

Cooking healthy with the Rice Diet doesn't require anything expensive or fancy. You'll just need the items on this list, many of which you probably have already:

- Measuring spoons and measuring cups
- A large measuring cup with handles (when appropriate for microwave use)
- A food scale or postal scale (measures in ounces up to a pound)
- Rice cooker
- Microwave
- Full set of microwave dishes (8 inches)
- Microwave steaming bags
- Blender
- Chopsticks (optional, but try them—they can help slow your eating down)

RICE CONGEE: WHAT IT IS, HOW TO MAKE IT

Rice congee, a staple of the Rice Diet, is also a staple in many Asian countries, where it is favored for its versatility in cooking and its healthful properties. It is essentially rice porridge (although not in granular form) that can be made to virtually any consistency. Rice congee has many benefits, including:

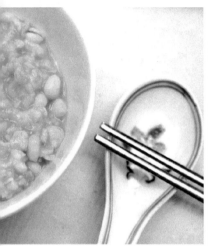
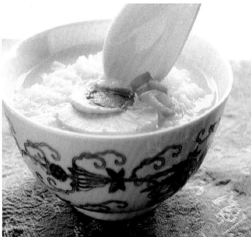

- Congee is a neutral tasting dish that works well with varied preparations
- Congee is a very light yet very filling dish
- A bowl of congee has far fewer calories than a bowl of plain rice (depending on how much water is added)
- The Rice Diet congee uses white rice or brown rice, both of which are low in sodium
- Congee can be mixed with vegetables, chicken or fish to make delicious meals
- Congee can be made in any consistency, from soup to pudding or thicker
- Congee can be eaten for breakfasts, lunches and dinners
- Congee can be flavored with many tasty, low-sodium spices

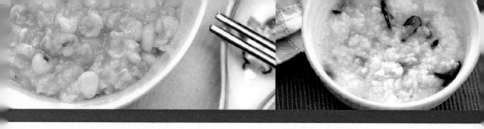

THREE METHODS OF MAKING CONGEE

The following is the authentic stove top method of cooking congee. Wash the rice, drain, and repeat until the water is clear. The amount of water you use depends upon the consistency desired. There are basically three rice to water ratios for different consistencies:

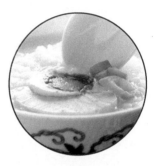

Thick: 1 cup rice to 8 cups water;
Medium: 1 cup rice to 10 cups water;
Thin: 1 cup rice to 13 cups water

Add the desired amount of water to the washed rice grains. Bring the water and rice to a boil before lowering the heat. Stir continuously to prevent the rice from sticking together or to the bottom of the pot. Stirring is important because rice grains, being much heavier than water, will settle to the bottom and stick to the pot. The disadvantage of cooking on the stove top is that you must consistently keep an eye on the congee for the entire cooking process, which is approximately 1.5 – 2 hours. Consider purchasing a rice cooker to make the process easier every time you wish to cook up a large quantity of congee to have for many meals.

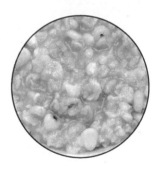

EXERCISE

Exercise is a key component of the Rice Diet. Exercise can speed metabolism, burn fat and increase muscle mass, plus it can help you lose weight without starving yourself. Chapter Four of this book discusses exercise in greater detail, but here we'll give you a brief introduction, beginning with this non-negotiable requirement:

Consult your physician for advice and approval before beginning any exercise regimen as part of your Rice Diet. Are we clear? Okay.

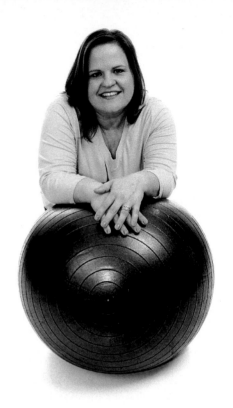

There are three activity levels established by the U.S. Department of Agriculture, to help determine how many calories you should consume daily:

Sedentary: Lifestyle includes only light physical activity associated with typical day-to-day life

Moderately Active: Includes physical activity equivalent to walking about 1.5 to 3 miles per day at 3 to 4 miles per hour; or, 30 to 60 minutes per day of moderate physical activity, in addition to daily activities

Active: 60 or more minutes per day of moderate physical activity in addition to daily activities

Obviously, your activity level should correspond to your physical ability and your doctor's recommendations, but the bottom line is: exercise is necessary to achieve success on the Rice Diet.

There is no specific set of exercises or exercise regimens required by the Rice Diet; you are basically free to create your own program in consultation with your doctor. However, one activity is always popular with Ricers:

WALKING

That's right, good old walking. It's a great form of exercise: it's easy to do, it doesn't cost much or require expensive gym memberships, and it can easily be done alone, with friends, and with other dieters. In recent years, "10,000-steps-a-day" has become an exercise routine for many Americans (more about that in Chapter Four). Should daily walking become your exercise of choice, you'll need:

• Comfortable exercise clothing
• Comfortable walking shoes
• A pedometer, a device that counts your steps as you walk (this is just our suggestion)

No matter what type of exercise you engage in, we strongly encourage you to embrace physical activity for weight loss, increased energy, stress relief, overall better health—and of course, for fun.

READY, SET, GO

Once you've consulted your doctor and purchased the required utensils and equipment, you're ready to live the Rice Diet lifestyle. You'll find recipes, menus, a weekly guide to the diet and more in Part Two of this book. As you begin your diet, it's important to consider some of the challenges you'll face in "staying with it"—and how to successfully meet them. We'll discuss these issues in the following chapters.

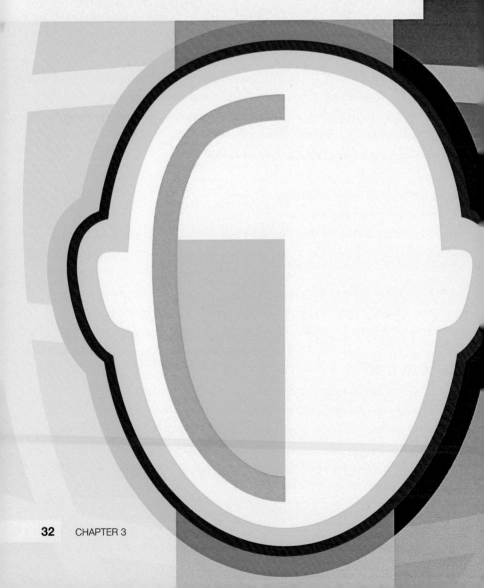

CHAPTER THREE
LOSING WEIGHT IS ALL IN YOUR HEAD

"People often say that motivation doesn't last. Well, neither does bathing—that's why we recommend it daily. "

\- Zig Ziglar

CHANCES ARE, YOU'RE NO STRANGER TO DIETING. If you've tried other diets and failed, you've probably told yourself, "I just can't lose weight." Well, here's good news: YOU'RE WRONG! The fact is, 99% of all obesity is not due to glandular problems, but to ingesting too many calories and getting too little exercise. It's as simple as that. These problems are fixable with the right program, the right motivation and the right approach. The Rice Diet is the right program, so let's look at the other two variables— motivation and approach.

IT STARTS WITH MOTIVATION: MIND OVER MATTERS

Losing weight isn't just a physical challenge. It's a mental challenge, too. And when it comes to the mental aspect of weight loss, we can be our own worst enemies—or our own best friends.

One key way to arm yourself in the fight to lose weight is through proper motivation. If you think you can't possibly summon the motivation to commit to the Rice Diet…think again. Every single day, you do things that prove you're one heck of a motivated person! For example, you get up in the morning and go to work or school. Motivation: a paycheck or a diploma. You come home and do the dishes, clean the house and throw out the trash. Motivation: a nicer, cleaner home. You try to save a little money each month from your income. Motivation: the security of having money for a rainy day. And on and on and on.

Now that we've dispelled the silly notion that you're not a motivated person, let's see how you can motivate yourself to commit to your diet and enjoy all the benefits of losing weight. A good place to start is by acknowledging that:

Losing weight is not always easy—but nothing worth having in life comes easy!

Ironically, admitting that weight loss doesn't just come with a snap of your fingers is the beginning of your motivation. Acknowledging this simple truth puts everything else in perspective. Like most activities in life, weight loss takes some effort and discipline. Some days are better than others, but if you stick with the program, you'll achieve the results you're seeking.

Try This Tip—Make a list of your accomplishments, great or small, and the things you did to achieve them. Examples:

ACCOMPLISHMENT	WORK REQUIRED
A+ in high school English	Lots of study; extra credit
Getting a promotion at work	Develop new ways to improve efficiency
Buying a new home	Economizing and budgeting to save money for a down payment

Keep this list handy. It's firsthand proof that diligent work and effort have paid off in your life—and a reminder that this same effort will pay off in your diet.

Now that you understand the work and rewards of dieting—and that **YOU CAN DO THIS**—the next step is to:

COMMIT TO YOUR RICE DIET IN WRITING

That's right, sign on the dotted line. Putting your commitment in writing is a powerful, tangible reminder that you recognize the importance of losing weight and living healthy, and that you take responsibility for making it happen. Think of it as a contract with yourself. And while this contract isn't legally binding, it may be the most important one you ever sign. This is your pledge to fight the good fight, to summon all your strength and determination so that excess weight will never steal another day, another moment of happiness from your life!

Do this now—You'll find the Contract to Commit To Living A New Lifestyle in Part Two (Chapter 16) of this book. Turn to it, read it, sign it—and commit to it.

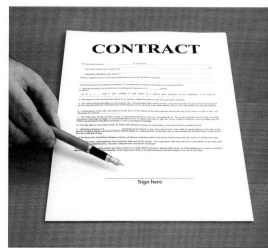

You can never have enough positive motivation in life, and one great way to build your own motivation is to:

SEEK INSPIRATION FROM OTHERS

Inspiration doesn't always come from within; sometimes we need someone or something to ignite the spark to inspire us. Albert Schweitzer put it very wisely: "In everyone's life, at some time, our inner fire goes out. It is then burst into flame by an encounter with another human being. We should all be thankful for those people who rekindle the inner spirit." The world is full of inspiring figures, historical and contemporary, who have faced challenges, battled adversity and won. You can draw from their strength and make it your own. And while you're at it, remember: YOU can become an inspiring figure to others as you succeed in losing weight, living healthier and changing your life. In other words, aspire to inspire!

Many behavior modification activities are easier when shared with others, such as quit-smoking classes at the local hospital. With this in mind, we suggest:

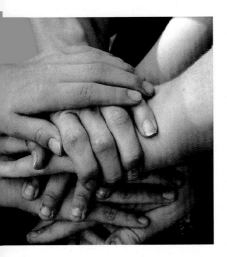

DIETING WITH OTHERS ON THE RICE DIET

Get a friend who wants to lose weight to join you on the Rice Diet. Or visit our Web site, www.ricedietcf.com. The understanding and encouragement you can receive from other Ricers can make a tremendous difference in the quality and success of your own diet.

Now, here's a little trick straight from Motivation 101:

REWARD YOURSELF FOR GOOD DIETING BEHAVIOR

There should be a fun component to dieting, and what could be more fun than rewarding yourself for taking responsibility and sticking with your program? So go ahead, buy something nice for yourself, or treat yourself to a spa massage, when you lose your first ten pounds. Then, when you've lost enough weight to fit into a smaller clothing size, take pleasure in buying a nice, new wardrobe as "a fitting way to celebrate" your achievement. Get creative, have fun (so long as you're not "treating" yourself with diet-breaking food!). You deserve it.

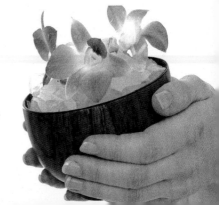

Dieting really is all about you. No one can do it for you. But with the right motivation, using some of these techniques along with others, you can take control of your diet, your weight, your health and your life. As you begin to control your eating and your weight, you'll notice a positive change in your ability to take charge of other aspects of your life. The sense of accomplishment you'll get will do wonders for your confidence and sense of self-worth. There's a snowball effect in all this, and once you get rolling, you'll be unstoppable!

MOTIVATIONAL POEM—DON'T QUIT

When things go wrong, as they sometimes will,
when the road you're trudging seems all up hill,
when the funds are low and the debts are high,
and you want to smile but you have to sigh,
when care is pressing you down a bit - rest if you must,
but don't you quit.
Life is queer with its twists and turns.
As every one of us sometimes learns.
And many a failure turns about when he might have won had he stuck it out.
Don't give up though the pace seems slow - you may succeed with another blow.
Often the goal is nearer than it seems to a faint and faltering man;
often the struggler has given up when he might have captured the victor's cup;
and he learned too late when the night came down,
how close he was to the golden crown.
Success is failure turned inside out - the silver tint of the clouds of doubt,
and you never can tell how close you are,
it may be near when it seem so far;
so stick to the fight when you're hardest hit - it's when things seem worse,
that you must not quit.

- Author of "Don't Quit" is unknown

KEEP YOUR COMMITMENT BY KEEPING A RICE DIET JOURNAL

As we mentioned before (and will continue to mention throughout this book), the Number-One most important thing in losing weight and changing your life is STAYING WITH THE PROGRAM. If you remain 100% committed to your Rice Diet plan, you can surely reach your goals. There are many ways to stay committed, such as the motivational techniques we just discussed. Another indispensable tool is the Rice Diet Journal, your own personal chronicle of your amazing journey from obesity to "Oh, what a great life I have!" Your journal

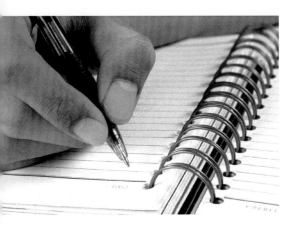

will become your ally, a "friend" that can help you begin to understand eating behavior and how to deal with it.

The first purpose of your journal is to keep track of what you eat and drink every day. Whenever you eat or drink something, whether a meal or a snack (or a nibble!), you'll record the amount you consumed and the time you consumed it. You'll also record daily weights, blood pressure, hunger level before eating, and how you felt after eating. We can't stress enough how important it is to be faithful and accurate in recording your eating habits, so:

Be sure to record every single eating event in your journal, right down to the smallest snack—even sampling food at the store or taking food off someone else's plate!

Your journal can provide a gold mine of valuable information about your eating habits, information you and your doctor can use to modify your eating routines, spot and correct bad eating behavior and otherwise help you become a healthier, "more successful" eater. But all these fantastic results can only happen if your journal is completely precise and truthful.

You will also record your exercise events in your journal, which will primarily consist of walking. Write in the time and distance of each walk you take, and, if you buy a pedometer, you can even record the number of steps taken!

SAMPLE JOURNAL

You'll find a sample Rice Diet Journal in Chapter 16. You may download a template of this user-friendly journal at **www.ricedietcf.com** or use the template to create your journal in a notebook. No matter which you choose, just remember: fill in your journal daily!

SHARE YOUR THOUGHTS AND FEELINGS

It's no secret that our emotions can have a tremendous effect, for good or bad, on our eating habits. Stress, anger, depression and even happiness can trigger seemingly uncontrollable urges to overeat. For this reason, there's a section in your journal for you to express your thoughts, feelings and emotions as they relate to your eating and to life in general. Chronicling your emotional state is certainly an excellent cathartic exercise, allowing you to vent, let off steam and diffuse emotions that are eating you up inside. Just as importantly, journaling about your emotional state can yield important insights about the things that cause you to eat unhealthily. Could it be boredom? Loneliness? Frustration? Journaling can help you confront these issues and motivate you to resolve them.

As with the other sections of your journal, it is important to be forthright when writing about your thoughts and emotions. This doesn't mean you have to beat yourself up or drag yourself down.

Instead, it simply means being honest about how you feel—and why. As you begin to accumulate entries in your journal, go over them, compare them, analyze them, and benefit from what you learn about yourself. With the Rice Diet, journaling isn't just a frivolous activity to pass away the hours. Years and years of experience have shown that journaling is a powerful aid in helping Rice Dieters conquer their weight problems.

In today's world, we often eat thoughtlessly, grabbing a quick bite here or there, getting a candy bar from the office vending machine or raiding the fridge before we go to bed. Journaling makes us more accountable for our eating behavior because it requires us to think about what we put into our mouths, whether or not it's good for us, or if we truly need it. Journaling also lets us examine and explore our feelings, which are almost always the root cause of our behavioral problems. Each page in your journal is a step towards your liberation, your freedom from the weight of obesity and medical problems, and the weight of unhappiness you presently live with.

They say the pen is mightier than the sword. We say the pen is mightier than the fork and knife! Let journaling be one of your powerful allies in your fight against obesity.

"BU-BU-BUT...I DON'T HAVE TIME TO WRITE A JOURNAL"

Ah, excuses, excuses. We've heard them all. But most of them aren't credible. Don't have time to keep a journal of the foods you consume? Well, every day you make grocery lists, shopping lists, to-do lists and so forth. How much different or more complicated is it to list the foods you eat? And you don't have to make your journal War and Peace. Many of the entries can be filled in quickly and easily. Look at it this way: a few minutes of journaling each day can help you enjoy an entire lifetime of health and happiness. Now that's a bargain! Journaling will also take the place of mindless eating. Put the fork down and pick up your pen instead!

Here's another excuse (typically from men): "Journals are for high school girls." Oh really? Well, hard-charging Teddy Roosevelt kept a diary. So did General George Patton, President Ronald Reagan and lots of other manly men. It doesn't matter whether you're a guy or a gal, or whether you can write like Shakespeare or not. The point is to take the thoughts and emotions inside you, the ones that are causing you to overeat—and get them outside your head by putting them on paper. You'll be amazed at how good it feels to do this. But just as important, the things you learn about yourself, such as your emotional triggers, can lead to effective solutions to your weight problems. Socrates said, "Know thyself." Allow us to amend that to, "Know thyself, and learn how to overcome obesity. Journal!"

As we mentioned, you always have choices in life. And in this case, you can choose to make excuses—or you can choose to make an effort. Which choice will cause you to lose weight and gain the life you've always dreamed of?

MANY PEOPLE THINK, 'WHY WRITE IN A JOURNAL? I'm the only one who's ever going to read it. Who cares what I have to say?' But the act of writing and reading what you've written can be very healing, especially if you're someone who struggles to identify what you're feeling or why you're feeling it. Journal writing is a great tool in learning to better understand your emotions and define what you're struggling with and what's bothering you.

—Amy Ojerhol, PhD, clinical psychologist

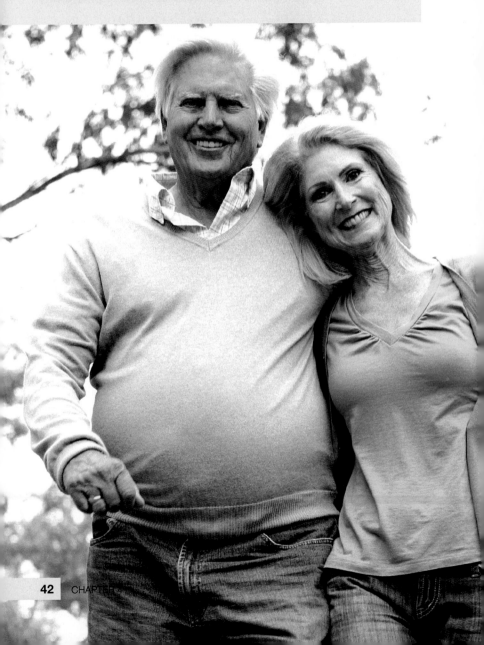

CHAPTER FOUR
EXERCISE YOUR RIGHT TO HEALTH AND HAPPINESS

"Those who think they have not time for bodily exercise will sooner or later have to find time for illness."

—Edward Stanley, Earl of Derby

WHY DO YOU SUPPOSE WE WERE PUT HERE ON EARTH? You could pose this question to a hundred different people and get a hundred different answers. But there's one thing all of us would agree on: We sure as heck weren't put here to be unhappy and unfulfilled in our lives! Each of us is driven to achieve some form of happiness, and we should all strive to improve ourselves. One timeless and universal method for improving our mental and physical state is through exercise.

When we say exercise, we're not talking about extreme or intense exertion. Instead, we're talking about ordinary, easily doable activities such as walking. It's been shown that walking as little as 10 minutes a day has a beneficial effect on one's physical and mental well-being, making it an ideal activity for anyone, especially those who wish to improve their health through weight loss. And yes, exercise is a must-do on the Rice Diet program.

It's not our purpose to create a specific exercise regimen for you. That's something you should probably do in partnership with your doctor, who knows your medical conditions and can help you tailor an exercise routine that's most appropriate for your capabilities and your goals. Instead, let us give you some general guidelines that will show you how exercise fits in with your diet, and how you can incorporate it into your life.

JACK LALANNE'S THOUGHTS ON DIET AND EXERCISE

Jack LaLanne was an American icon of fitness, exercise and nutrition. These zingers from Jack are worth sharing—and remembering:

"Exercise is king, nutrition is queen. Put them together and you've got a kingdom!"

"Eat right and you can't go wrong."

"Your waistline is your lifeline."

"Your health account is like your bank account—the more you put in, the more you can take out."

DIET AND EXERCISE, THE RICE DIET WAY

In one sense, the Rice Diet is a balancing act, because it's really about getting your life in balance. Exercise speeds your metabolism and burns fat, helping "consume" the calories from what you eat. Think of a balance scale, with one side representing calories, and the other representing exercise to burn off those calories. With the right amount of each, your body is in balance. Exercise also has a very positive effect on your emotional health, and this is another dimension of the balance we need to achieve. In addition to strengthening your body and lifting your spirits, exercise can help firm your character by demanding commitment and rewarding you with a sense of accomplishment. Exercise is good for you in every aspect of your well being.

One last thing: regular exercise can let you eat more food without weight gain—that means you can enjoy more tasty, healthy Rice Diet dishes without guilt. What a deal!

MAKE IT MANAGEABLE

No one's asking you to sign up for a triathlon in the first week of your diet! In fact, overdoing exercise is not good for anyone's health. What you need to do is develop an exercise routine you can manage, and benefit from, daily. We strongly recommend consulting your doctor about this. Your goal here isn't to create a laundry list of exercises (borr-ing!). Rather, you'll want to create a routine that's 100% tailored to your needs, capabilities and goals for good health. As you learn more about physical activity, you'll see there are endless ways to get—and stay—in shape. Many of these activities, such as stretching and breathing exercises, are simple ones that you can easily integrate into your everyday routine.

DO IT DAILY

Daily exercise is something everyone should do, and if you're a Ricer, it's something you really must do. First, you won't get the full benefits of exercise—weight loss, improved health, feeling good physically and emotionally—if you only exercise occasionally. It just doesn't work that way. The calories that go into your body don't get burned off by watching TV or sitting at your computer all day. You gotta keep moving if you wanna keep losing.

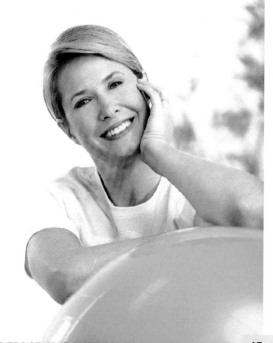

Exercising daily is also easier on you—literally. As your muscles become accustomed to use (and they will in short order), they'll expect and even look forward to their daily walk, or whatever exercise you engage them in. Slack off for a few days, and those happy, eager muscles of yours will revert to their previous unused state. Then you'll have to start all over again—and your muscles, grumpy over their inactivity, will get back at you with aches and pains. If you want to make exercise more comfortable and easy on your body, you need to do it daily.

Of course, there will be days when you can't do your full exercise routine, such as when the weather doesn't cooperate. No problem. You can still do something, such as seeking out indoor malls (no stopping at the food court, just walk!), taking the stairs to your office or just walking around your house. Some exercise is better than none, and while your goal should always be to do your established exercise program every day, don't let bad weather (or anything) be an excuse for doing nothing.

MAKE IT FUN

Exercising can be fun! That's a main theme of the Rice Diet. And let us assure you, there's no lack of fun ways to enjoy physical activity on a daily basis. Most cities and towns have numerous parks, walking paths, or interesting sites you can reach on foot. Become an explorer and experience them. Remember too that many of the activities you think of as fun can also be great exercise opportunities. Gardening, washing your car, dancing, walking around while talking on your phone—these are just some of the things you can do that can also be part of your exercise routine.

While you're at it, why not share the fun? Walk with a friend or get involved in an exercise group with people who have similar goals to yours. Exercising with others is a great way to stay motivated and focused. It's also rewarding in a social sense, since you're sharing a good, healthy activity with like-minded people. This sharing and camaraderie can have a wonderfully positive impact not only on your diet, but on the quality of your relationships as well.

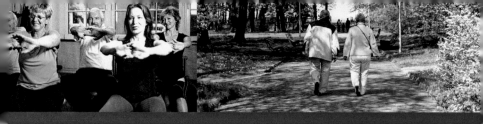

EXERCISE IS YOUR FRIEND!

The benefits of exercising are truly amazing and almost endless. Obviously, exercise helps control your weight. It also builds and strengthens muscles, including your heart. Exercise helps ward off illness and disease, including depression, anxiety and other debilitating illnesses. Exercise gives you energy and boosts your sense of well-being. There is increasing clinical evidence that shows the moderating effects of exercise on the aging process, including everything from controlling arthritis pain to reducing the possibility of dementia or Alzheimer's. And all it takes to enjoy these benefits are some comfortable clothing, a pair of walking shoes and a pedometer. Exercise is one of the greatest gifts to humankind. Take advantage of this gift, and enjoy!

REGULAR EXERCISE CAN NOT ONLY HELP YOU LOSE WEIGHT BUT...

- Reduce your risk of dying from heart disease or stroke
- Lower risk of heart disease, stroke, high blood pressure, colon cancer and diabetes
- Protect against bone fractures in older adults
- Help protect against breast cancer
- Help keep your bones, muscles and joints healthy
- Reduce anxiety and depression
- Help you handle stress
- Help control joint swelling and pain from arthritis
- Help you feel more energetic
- Help you sleep better
- Help formulate a routine and a sense of purpose
- Help increase self-esteem and confidence

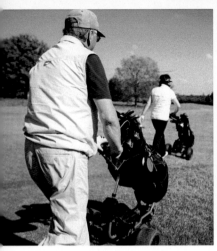
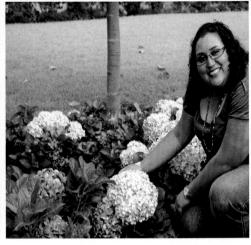

TIP TOP SHAPE: EIGHT TIPS

1 **Plan to stay in shape**—Start by planning a realistic exercise program, preferably with your doctor. Together, you can determine the types of exercise best suited for your medical conditions and your weight loss goals. Developing a plan gives structure to your exercise routine, making it easier to follow—and easier to succeed. Developing a plan with your doctor assures that your exercise regimen is tailored to your needs and capabilities.

2 **Do more when you're ready and able**—You may outgrow your beginning exercise regimen as you become stronger and more fit. You should then add to your regimen: a few more minutes of walking, a few more calisthenics, a few more laps of the pool. Consult your doctor, but don't shy away from stepping up your program. It's good for you.

3 **Anywhere, anytime**—Anytime you're moving, you're exercising. Walk around the room when you're on the phone. Get up and out of your office regularly to stretch and take a few steps. Create opportunities to do something instead of nothing, such as:
- Marching in place while you're watching the morning news on TV
- Moving your arms and legs when sitting in a chair
- Installing a treadmill in your home and using it regularly

4 **Don't get discouraged by minor aches and pains** — These small discomforts, experienced by most people when they start exercising, are telling you that your exercise is working! Your muscles are waking up, getting accustomed to use, and after a short period of time, the aches and pains will be gone, and in their place will be a healthier you!

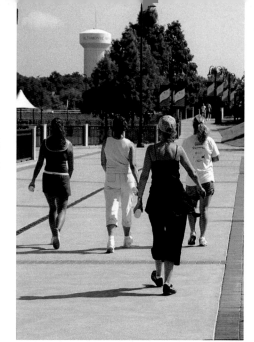

5 **Seek motivation and encouragement** — Staying with a program of regular exercise isn't always easy, even for lifelong devotees of physical fitness. If you feel your motivation flagging, discuss it with your doctor, good friends, or others you know who can give you encouragement. You can also recharge your motivational batteries by learning the stories of others who have faced and conquered adversity. On the Internet, greatday.com offers a wealth of motivational material and resources that you can access quite easily.

While you alone are ultimately responsible for your exercise program, you don't have to do it alone. There are many people and resources that can help encourage and motivate you. Use them!

6 **Exercise with others** — This, in combination with Tip 4, may be your best way to maintain daily motivation and encouragement. We strongly recommend it for anyone, particularly those with severe weight problems. Exercise with a friend, a fellow worker, a neighbor or others who are similarly committed to good health, or join a fitness club or center. Studies have shown that quitting smoking with others dramatically improves one's own chance for success. The same principle applies to exercise and weight loss.

7 **Become an exercise expert**—This doesn't mean you have to get a PhD in kinesiology or sports medicine. Just take the time to learn about your favorite exercises and how to maximize your enjoyment of them. If you walk, for example, read up on the subject, join a walking group, explore all the interesting walks in your city or region, etc. What we're suggesting here is that you turn your exercise program into your hobby, or even your passion. This can really add to the fun and satisfaction you get from your activity. Every time you exercise, you'll feel better physically and mentally, and experience a sense of accomplishment as well.

8 **If you already have an exercise regimen ... keep doing it!**

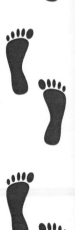

10,000 STEPS A DAY KEEPS THE DOCTOR AWAY
A number of recent medical studies suggest that walking 10,000 steps a day is a good "ballpark number" for maintaining health and fitness. Sound like a lot? Well, consider that even the average sedentary person walks up to 3,000 steps a day. Getting up to 10,000 a day then is not impossible. With a pedometer, you can track your daily steps. Determine your present number of steps as a baseline and then work up to 10,000. Doing this should take you no more than 30 minutes per day, which you can break up into three 10-minute walking periods if you like. Get in your 10,000 steps a day, and you might just end up walking away from obesity and its inherent health problems.

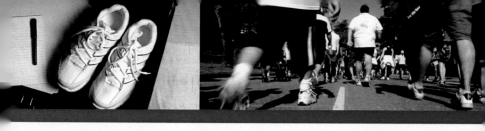

BURN CALORIES AT WORK

Small changes in your routine can help you burn calories around the office.

Typical day at the office (calories burned)
Park by building, take elevator to floor (15)
Make phone calls for an hour at desk (15)
Seated 45-minute lunch (25)
Seated 1-hour meeting (15)
Take elevator to ground floor, walk to car, drive home (15)

Total (85 calories burned)

Picking up the pace (calories burned)
Park 5 blocks from office, take stairs to floor (80-120)
Take calls standing up and pacing (100-130)
Walk 30 minutes at lunch, sit and eat 15 minutes (100-130)
1-hour walking meeting (150-200)
Take stairs out of building, walk back to car (80-120)

Total (510-680 calories burned)

Bottom Line
Sit less, stand more, move more, lose more.

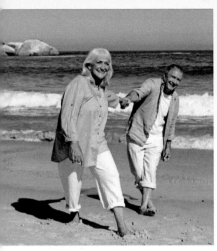
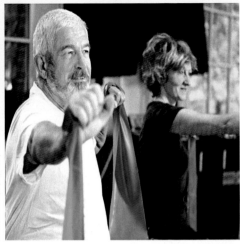

"I CAN'T WALK TODAY BECAUSE (INSERT FAVORITE EXCUSE HERE)"
Sorry, but excuses don't help you lose weight, shed your obesity and transform your life. Only exercise does that. Yes, there are legitimate reasons and times for not exercising, and any reasonable person can recognize and understand them. But "legitimate reason" and "excuse" are not the same thing! In one sense, exercise is a physical activity that strengthens your body, but the act of committing to exercise, and following through, is a mental activity that builds up your will, your resolve and your character. This is every bit as important as the purely physical benefits you get from exercise; having firm character will help you immensely at succeeding with your diet, and of course, in many other areas of your life. Let your motto then be: Exercise, Not Excuses!

What's your excuse for not walking? Stop making excuses and start making progress!

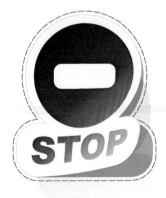

EXERCISE, AND BECOME AN EX-OBESE PERSON!

We exercise and we know many, many other people who do too. It's easier for some than others. Some people are workout fanatics, while others stick to a daily walk or a jog. But there's one thing they all agree on: exercise makes their lives better. They feel happier, more relaxed, more energetic—in a word, healthier. Whatever small price they pay in commitment, time, the occasional aches and pains and so forth, is amply repaid by the joy of feeling fit.

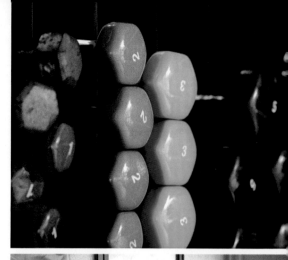

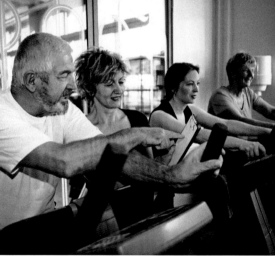

And the overwhelming majority of these people aren't bodybuilders or triathletes, they're just regular people who regularly exercise. This includes many people who used to be overweight or even obese. Thanks to the Rice Diet, they overcame their inertia, they dropped the excuses, they assumed responsibility for their health, and they took action. Why not you?

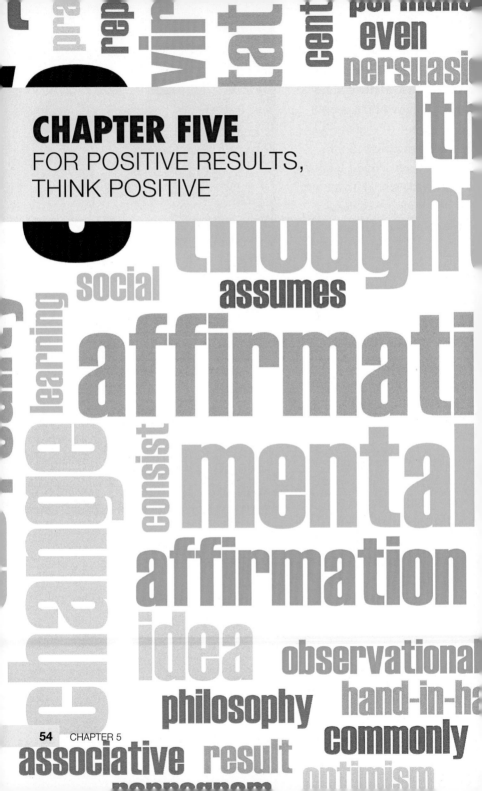

CHAPTER FIVE
FOR POSITIVE RESULTS, THINK POSITIVE

> *"A person will be just about as happy as they make up their mind to be."*
>
> —Abraham Lincoln

ABRAHAM LINCOLN'S THOUGHTS ON HOW TO BE HAPPY—by setting one's mind to it—are pretty much at the core of the Rice Diet. As we now know, dieting is about how we think as well as how we eat, and a positive frame of mind is essential for success.

For many people, achieving and maintaining a consistently positive attitude is a challenge. After all, life is not always easy, it's not always a piece of cake—and neither is dieting (especially the cake part!). If you have a serious weight problem, it surely diminishes your sense of happiness, and this only contributes to your reliance on food as a source of gratification and comfort. It sounds like a vicious circle, but this circle can be broken. It will take time, effort, practice and patience, but the fact is, just as the human mind becomes conditioned to unhappiness and negativity, it can also be directed (trained, if you will) to think positively, embrace challenge and change, and triumph over any of the obstacles life throws in our paths.

History is filled with endless examples of people who have persevered and overcome, largely though faith in themselves and a belief that through taking action, they would triumph over adversity. Sure, some of these people were simply extraordinary human beings, maybe a cut above you and the rest of us. But the overwhelming majority were just regular folks, people who had the same doubts, insecurities and fears of failure that most of us have. Oftentimes, these people were backed into a corner where they had little choice but to think positively, remain optimistic under the most difficult circumstances, and take action. The key word in that last sentence is "choice"—they made the choice to think positive and remain optimistic. That is what we all must do.

In this chapter, we'll explore positive thinking as it relates to your Rice Diet program, and we'll also discuss ways to create and maintain an optimistic attitude. Please, don't just commit to positive thinking — **embrace it with all your heart and soul**; it is your Great Liberator, the irresistible power within you that can free you from obesity and to live the life you dream of!

"THINK POSITIVE" BY NORMAN VINCENT PEALE

If you want to get somewhere, you have to know where you want to go,
and how to get there.
Then never, never, never give up.
The secret of life isn't what happens to you,
but what you do with what happens to you.
Help other people to cope with their problems
and your own will be easier to cope with.
Never use the word impossible seriously again.
Toss it into the verbal wastebasket.
Self-trust is the first secret of success.
So believe in and trust yourself.
Stand up to your obstacles and do something about them.
You will find that they haven't half the strength you think they have.
Joy increases as you give it,
and diminishes as you try to keep it for yourself.
In giving it, you will accumulate a deposit of joy
greater than you ever believed possible.
How you think about a problem is more important
than the problem itself — so always think positively.
Go at life with abandon; give it all you've got.
And life will give all it has to you.

THE TRUTH WILL SET YOU FREE

A good place to start our journey to becoming a positive person is by acknowledging some fundamental truths. Not all of these truths are pleasant, but by facing them directly and without fear, we get a true picture of our situation, and how to overcome it.

Truth: Dieting is not easy—Okay, we've already said this, and you already understand it. But it bears repeating. Dieting requires a change in behavior, and this doesn't happen overnight. Along the way, there are triumphs and setbacks, good days and bad. Results don't come instantly, and they require effort and commitment. There is frustration and discouragement along with the joys and triumphs.

Truth: Neither is dieting impossible—You've heard this before as well, but we want to make sure it sinks in. As we've said, 99% of all obesity comes from overeating. This is actually cause for optimism, because it means virtually all obesity is reversible, fixable. By following your Rice Diet regimen, you can lose weight. By sticking with it, you can keep that weight off.

Truth: You are not alone in your battle against obesity—As you read this, there are many other seriously overweight people in your area (and virtually everywhere) who are determined to lose weight and transform their lives. Seek them out for support and understanding. Our Web site, ricedietcf.com, is another great resource for support. Sharing the ups and downs of dieting with other dieters is tremendously helpful and increases your chances of long-term success.

Truth: A setback is a setback, not defeat—There is no such thing as a "perfect" dieter. We all experience

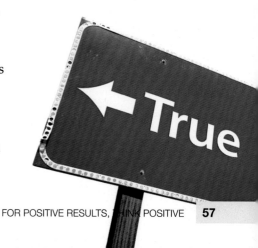

setbacks and slip-ups, whether it's failing to exercise or eating the wrong foods. Just as we choose to do these things, we can also choose to get back on our diet. So, after a setback, don't beat yourself up or give in to despair. Learn from your mistakes, so you don't make them again. Get back on your exercise/diet program with your next meal or your next scheduled walk. Also, use your setback as an opportunity to learn (this is where your journal is invaluable). What triggered the setback? How could you have handled it differently? What can you do to avoid this situation in the future? The more you understand about your setbacks, the better you'll understand how to succeed.

Truth: Positive thinking succeeds. YOU are a positive person—If you're obese, you may not feel too positive right now, but trust us, that positivity is in you just waiting to be unleashed. We know this because—well, you're reading this book. That tells us you do believe there's an answer out there to your weight problem, and if you find it, you do believe you can lose weight. The fact that you've chosen the Rice Diet tells us you're not only a positive person—but pretty darn smart, too.

TAKE A REALITY CHECK

As you begin your journey to becoming a positive-thinking person, you should take time for a little introspection. How happy are you? What makes you happy? What makes you unhappy? What changes in your life, along with weight loss, might increase your happiness? Answering these questions honestly and without judgment can help you understand your problem and focus on solutions. It can also increase your motivation and your resolve to take action.

POINTERS ON POSITIVE THINKING AND ATTITUDE

There is a wealth of information on the subject of positive thinking available on the Internet, at bookstores and through your local library (we'll share some of our favorite books and resources later). Here, we'll give you some basic tools and skills for building and maintaining a positive attitude, techniques you can use every day to improve the quality of your diet and your life. Make any—or preferably all—of the following part of your daily routine:

Recite affirmations—Affirmations are simple statements about yourself, your abilities, your commitment to a goal and your determination to achieve it. You'll find a list of affirmations in Part Two of this book, but there's one you should say to yourself several times a day:

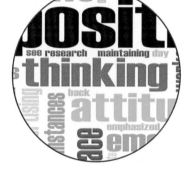

I can follow the Rice Diet regimen. I can lose weight and regain my health. I can dream, believe and achieve.

Memorize this, or post it on your refrigerator. Say it out loud and make it your mantra. Reciting affirmations such as this one is a good, simple way to train your mind to think positively. If you believe in yourself anything is possible—you can do it!

Journal your achievements and accomplishments—Write down the good things you do in your Rice Diet journal. Set a goal of doing at least one thing you feel good about every day, then record it in your journal. It doesn't matter whether your achievements are great or small; what's important is that you did them. Journaling your accomplishments gets you in the habit of striving for improvement, and it lets you see the connection between positive action and positive outcomes.

Think positive thoughts, banish negative ones—We almost cringe at writing something so obvious, but it's astounding how often (and easily) we let our minds succumb to unhealthy preoccupations. Such as how to deal with your difficult boss. Or steaming about the bad grade your teacher gave you when you didn't study for your science test. Don't let your mind get away with this! Instead, train it to focus on the good things in your life, such as family and friends, pets, hobbies and interests, and spiritual matters if you're religious or spiritually inclined. As Abe Lincoln said, make up your mind to be happy, and you will be.

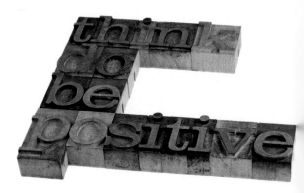

Think positive thoughts about your diet—Sure, dieting is hard. But rather than dwell on that, why not think about all the benefits you will reap from it. Fix your mind on your improved health, reversing your medical conditions, looking and feeling better, being more active and energetic, and on and on. That's bound to make you happy.

Change is good, so embrace it—It's not easy to break old habits, even the unhealthy ones we need to be rid of. However, you must be willing to change if you wish to succeed with your diet. Look at it this way: doing things your present way hasn't succeeded, so why not make some changes that could lead to success? You really have nothing to lose by trying (except your excess weight and your health problems!). As you make the changes called for in your diet, try other little things, like taking a different way to work or getting up 15 minutes earlier to do deep breathing exercises. Sometimes, changing your routine can help you get out of the rut you've been stuck in.

Enjoy positive activities with positive people—Obesity can make a person withdrawn, shunning healthy activities and company because of shame or humiliation. Solitude can be relaxing and restoring, but what we're talking about here is isolation—that's not good. As you know, we absolutely recommend sharing your Rice Diet lifestyle with others who are doing the same. And if there are any Negative Neds or Nancys in your life, avoid them in favor of people who 100% support and encourage your wonderful new life.

"DESIDERATA" BY MAX EHRMANN

Go placidly amid the noise and haste,
and remember what peace there may be in silence.
As far as possible without surrender be on good terms with all persons.
Speak your truth quietly and clearly; and listen to others,
even the dull and the ignorant; they too have their story.
Avoid loud and aggressive persons, they are vexations to the spirit.
If you compare yourself with others, you may become vain and bitter;
for always there will be greater and lesser persons than yourself.
Enjoy your achievements as well as your plans.
Keep interested in your own career, however humble;
it is a real possession in the changing fortunes of time.
Exercise caution in your business affairs; for the world is full of trickery.
But let this not blind you to what virtue there is;
many persons strive for high ideals;
and everywhere life is full of heroism.
Be yourself. Especially, do not feign affection.
Neither be cynical about love;
for in the face of all aridity and disenchantment
it is as perennial as the grass.
Take kindly the counsel of the years,
gracefully surrendering the things of youth.
Nurture strength of spirit to shield you in sudden misfortune.
But do not distress yourself with dark imaginings.
Many fears are born of fatigue and loneliness.
Beyond a wholesome discipline,
be gentle with yourself.
You are a child of the universe,
no less than the trees and the stars;
you have a right to be here.
And whether or not it is clear to you,
no doubt the universe is unfolding as it should.
Therefore be at peace with God, whatever you conceive Him to be,
and whatever your labors and aspirations,
in the noisy confusion of life keep peace with your soul.
With all its sham, drudgery, and broken dreams,
it is still a beautiful world. Be cheerful. Strive to be happy.

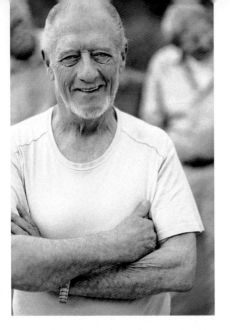

Don't "feed" your emotions—Anger, sadness, frustration, loneliness, depression. They can happen to anyone, even the most positive thinking person in the world. It's how you deal with these emotions that's important. First, know that eating doesn't resolve emotional issues (more about this in the next chapter). In fact, it only fuels them—and while food is "fuel," it should not be fuel for negative emotions! And the truth is, the emotional compensation we get from unhealthy eating is fleeting, and the pounds we add only increase our suffering and misery. Of course, there are many healthy, effective ways to deal with our emotional problems, including:

• Support groups and friends
• Spiritual leaders and counselors
• Creative activities such as writing in your Rice Diet journal
• Exercise

We all face challenges in life, but they can also create opportunities for personal growth and achievement. Remember this as you meet the challenges in your life.

Have an attitude of gratitude—No matter how adverse your situation is, can you honestly say you have nothing in life to be thankful for? Chances are, you have many things for which you can be grateful, from good parents and good friends down to simple things like a beautiful day or a favorite piece of music (remember, it's the simple, little things in life that are the big things). Gratitude is a great blessing, because it expresses our love of life and other people in a most genuine and unassuming way. It's also a tremendously potent antidote to negativity, because it washes the film of despair from our eyes and lets us see our life in a purer and truer light. Have an attitude of gratitude every day, and there will always be some good, even in your most trying days.

The Little Things
It really is the little things
That mean the most of all...
The "let me help you with that" things
That may seem very small
The "I'll be glad to do it" things
That make your cares much lighter,
The "laugh with me, it's funny" things
That make your outlook brighter...
The "never mind the trouble" things,
The "yes, I understand,"
The interest and encouragement
In everything you've planned
It really is the little things,
The friendly word or smile,
That add such happiness to life
And make it more worthwhile.
—*Mary Dawson Hughes*

> **Enjoy the little things,** for one day you may look back and realize they were the big things.
> - *Robert Brault*

Have some faith—If you are a religious person, draw on your faith for strength and power in your quest for good health. If you are not a religious or spiritual person, have faith in yourself—you are an exceptional person for making the decision to take charge of your life and take action to lose weight and regain your health. Even the smallest triumph, such as eating a piece of fruit for dessert, an apple instead of apple pie, is cause for you to say, "I can stay with my diet. I have just proven this. I have faith in myself."

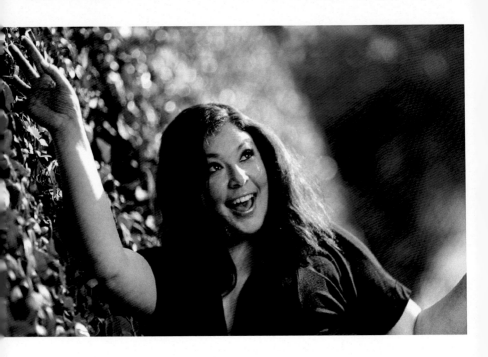

Go steady, Freddie—Developing a deeply rooted positive attitude doesn't happen overnight. Give yourself time, practice your attitude adjustment techniques, and plan to make steady progress in transforming your mental framework. Affirmations, journaling and grateful thoughts are things you can do from day one, while other things, such as finding a good support group, may require a bit more time and investigation. Don't get discouraged if you struggle with your transformation; it's not easy emerging from the cocoon of negativity to spread your wings. Talk with your doctor, counselor, friends, family or therapist as you go along, and let them be part of your "new attitude" plan. If you take a day-by-day approach to developing a positive attitude, and work at it every day, you'll experience a life-changing transformation over time. We're positive of that.

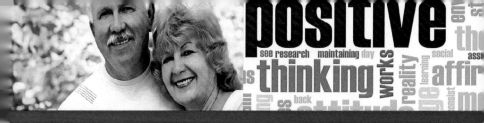

POSITIVE WORDS: CHOOSE 'EM AND USE 'EM

Take a word from this list each day and use it to complete the sentence:

Today I can be a(n) _____ person. Repeat the sentence to yourself several times during the day.

Active, Adventurous, Authentic, Awesome, Beautiful, Bold, Brave, Capable, Caring, Confident, Courageous, Curious, Dependable, Determined, Distinct, Dynamic, Energetic, Enthusiastic, Exceptional, Fascinating, Feisty, Fun, Gutsy, Happy, Hardworking, Healthy, Helpful, Honest, Imaginative, Important, Interesting, Intelligent, Joyful, Kind, Likeable, Lively, Loyal, Magical, Motivated, Memorable, Natural, Nice, Noticeable, Open-Minded, Optimistic, Original, Patient, Persistent, Positive, Precious, Proud, Quirky, Real, Reliable, Resourceful, 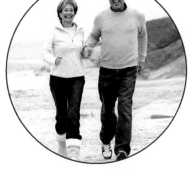 Responsible, Sharp, Smiley, Spiritual, Supportive, Surprising, Sympathetic, Thoughtful, Tolerant, Trustworthy, Unique, Unselfish, Unwavering, Upbeat, Valuable, Versatile, Vigorous, Vital, Warm, Willing, Wise, Witty, Wonderful.

THE HUMAN MIND: DON'T UNDERESTIMATE IT!

Is there anything more amazing, more astounding in the entire universe than the human mind? The power of the mind to dream, create, love, learn, imagine, reason, articulate—it's miraculous! But of course, all these good things don't happen by accident. As with so many things in life, we choose how to use our minds. We can think good thoughts, or bad. We can aspire to happiness and fulfillment in life, or resign ourselves to bitterness and defeat. The power of the mind is such that how we use it—the choices we make in employing it—largely determines our fate in life.

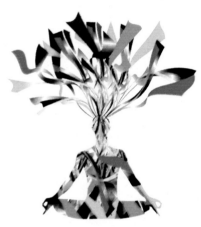

Knowing this, we ask: why would anyone choose negativity over the positive?

For goodness sake, cherish your mind, this gift beyond all gifts, and use it to be the happy, engaged, fulfilled and fully realized person you surely are meant to be. Team up with your mind to POSITIVELY fight and conquer your weight problem. If you work together, obesity doesn't stand a chance!

A BIT OF ZEN WISDOM

Once there was a college professor who wanted to learn the deepest, most profound truth of that mysterious religion, Zen Buddhism. So he went to Japan, visited a Zen monastery, and asked the head priest, "What is the deepest, most profound truth of your mysterious religion?" The priest replied, "Be a good person." "WHAT?" cried the professor, "I came all this way to hear that? Why, every six-year-old knows it's important to be a good person!"

"Yes," said the priest, "every six-year-old knows that—but how many of us actually do it?"

We share this story for those of you who wonder why we keep hammering on things like motivation, commitment and positive thinking. After all, we all know these are good things, right? Of course we do. But unless we practice them, our knowledge of these principles is for naught—and our diet goes down the tubes. So please, take all of the simple, obvious, "I knew that but needed to be reminded" stuff in this book and put it into practice in your daily life. Refer to this book over and over for reminders about the importance of doing the little things to achieve big things. Do this, and you'll attain your ideal weight—and a lot of other good things in life.

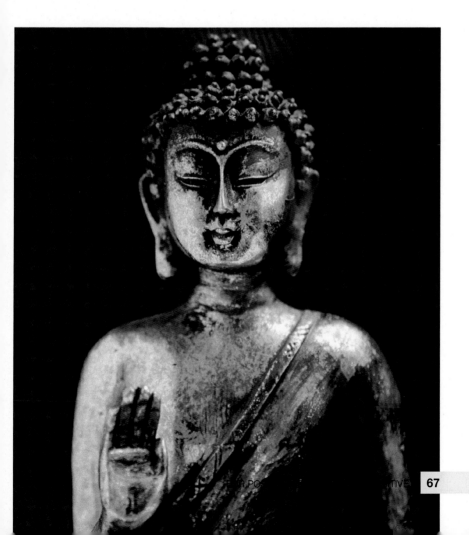

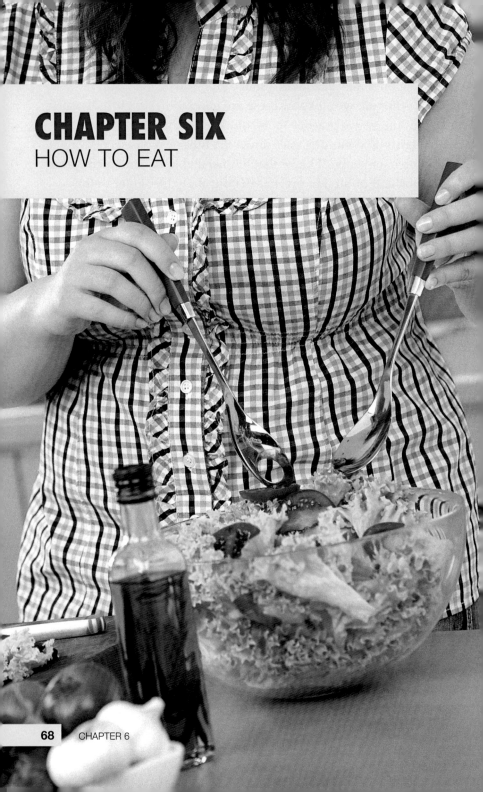

CHAPTER SIX
HOW TO EAT

"To lengthen thy life, lessen thy meals."
—Benjamin Franklin

TECHNICALLY SPEAKING, anyone who knows how to use a fork and knife (or chopsticks, for that matter) knows how to eat. Heck, you can even use your hands in a pinch. But the problem is, many of us don't know how to eat right—and by eating right, we're not only talking about what food we eat, but how we consume it. There really is an art and science to the consumption of food that, when practiced, causes us to be healthier, and to even enjoy our food more.

We may have learned some of these practices in our childhood, and simply forgotten or abandoned them over time. But we suspect a host of cultural influences are the real culprits here, encouraging and even teaching us bad habits of food consumption. We live in a frantically paced society that emphasizes instant gratification. We're bombarded with commercial messages that shout Bigger is Better. We turn to substances, be it drink, drugs or food, to "deal with" the stresses of modern life. In such an environment, it's no wonder we gobble foods high in sodium, fat and sugar, and yet receive no lasting benefit or satisfaction from them.

• Knowing how to properly consume food is essential for the success of your diet and health—and the quality of your life
• Consuming food as it is meant to be consumed will enhance your enjoyment of eating far beyond what you presently experience
• Practicing proper food consumption can positively affect other areas of your life, such as your self-discipline and mindfulness

Yes, it is possible to learn how to eat for health, nutrition and enjoyment. But this means a change in behavior, entirely abandoning our bad eating habits in favor of healthful ones. As we already know, changing behavior is not easy, requires effort and determination, and does not happen quickly. But if you follow your Rice Diet, food will become your friend, nourishing and sustaining you, instead of causing havoc in your life. Is following a simple diet too great a price to pay for a lifetime of health and happiness? We all know the answer to that.

LIVE TO EAT, EAT TO LIVE

What is the purpose of food? Is it a digestible form of happiness, comfort or relief from emotional turmoil? Absolutely not. Of course, we often use food in these ways, or should we say, misuse it. But the fundamental truth is:

Food is fuel for the body, providing nutrients and minerals which the body converts into energy to sustain life.

Simply put, we eat to live, and any diet that does not spring from this premise is flawed. We strongly suggest that you make "I eat to LIVE" one of your diet mantras. Put it on your refrigerator if you like. Use it to remind yourself that your body is a machine that requires proper dietary maintenance to run smoothly.

Now please, don't get the false impression that Eating to Live means boring eating. Not at all. On the Rice Diet, you can eat delicious and satisfying meals, snacks and foods. The only difference is, the tasty food you eat on the Rice Diet will actually be good for you, instead of harming you. Taste

EAT-TO-LIVE

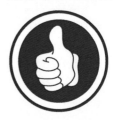

LIVE-TO-EAT

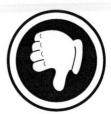

and yummynesswise (now there's a Scrabble word!), the Rice Diet will leave you full, satisfied, and saying to yourself, "Mmmm, that was good."

EATING 101

Learning how to eat to achieve and maintain your ideal weight is not rocket science. It requires some thought and self-discipline, but you'll be fine if you follow these rules, tips and suggestions:

Get a calorie counter book and use it—Our favorite book is Corrine T. Netzer's *The Complete Book of Food Counts*, which you can order through the Internet or a bookstore. No matter which book you select, make sure it includes fat, sugar and sodium content as well as calories.

Eat when you are physically hungry—For most people, real physical hunger occurs approximately 4-6 hours after the last eaten meal. A reliable sign of physical hunger is stomach growling. Get in the habit of eating your meals several hours apart, and know that if you feel hungry without any physical signs, you're probably experiencing emotional hunger—that is, phantom hunger—which shouldn't be fed.

Get rid of your unhealthy foods—And not by eating them, please! Whatever you do, rid your table, your shelves and your pantry of junk food snacks and the like, and replace them with fruits, vegetables and other healthy treats. Banish the junk, banish the temptation.

Go ahead, spoil your appetite—You know the old admonition, "Don't spoil your appetite by snacking between meals." Well, on the Rice Diet, snacking between meals is fine—so long as the snack is a piece of fruit or a vegetable. REPLACE the junk food snacks with a crisp, sweet apple or a banana. You'll be amazed at how quickly you'll come to prefer these healthy snacks.

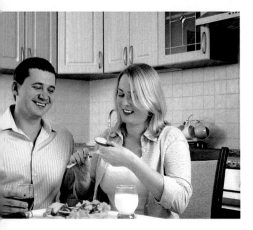

Eat slowly—Studies have shown that, in addition to causing indigestion, excess gas, belching and other problems, eating quickly causes people to overeat. So slow down a little. Cut your food into smaller bites and chew it thoroughly. Put your knife and fork down often during your meal to savor the taste of your food, take some sips of water and enjoy some table talk with your fellow diners. Instead of gobbling your meal down in a few minutes, take 15 or 20 minutes to eat (that's the amount of time it takes from your brain to "tell" your stomach it's full). You like to eat (we all do!), so why rush it? Eating slowly will help you eat less, and enjoy your meal more. It can even reduce your calorie intake!

Drink water, then eat—Many health care experts recommend drinking eight 8 oz. glasses of water per day, just for general health. Drinking 1-2 glasses of water before a meal is a healthy way to reduce your appetite and the amount of food you eat.

"The kitchen is closed"—Make it your nightly practice to eat no more after dinner, especially nothing in the two to three hours before you go to bed. Read a book, take a shower, listen to music, write a letter or send an e-mail—there are many things you can do in the evening besides nighttime nibbling, so do them!

Cook/store/eat—It's tempting to go for fast food and such when we come home to an empty fridge. A much better idea is to cook meals in large amounts, then store and freeze them in smaller containers, so they're ready for you when you need them. In the time it takes to go to a fast food place (or wait in the fast food line), you can enjoy a delicious, healthy meal in the comfort of your own home.

Every bite matters—Remember, sampling food at the grocery store or munching from a snack tray at a Super Bowl party counts as eating. Even little tastes of this and that can add to your daily caloric intake, which can mess up your diet. It's important to avoid these cheater treats.

WHOA! YOU'RE NOT A BOA!
Just about all of us are guilty of gulping down a meal from time to time, seemingly in one bite. But that doesn't make it right, or excuse the behavior. Go slow when you eat; it's better for your weight and your health.

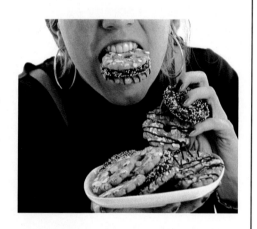

These are just a few of the many, many ways you can eat smarter, to lose weight and improve your health. We suggest—make that insist—that you take them to heart, and make them part of your daily eating habits.

Now, let's move on to the most important Eating 101 tip—the number one thing you can do to assure you're eating food in the most healthful, beneficial manner possible.

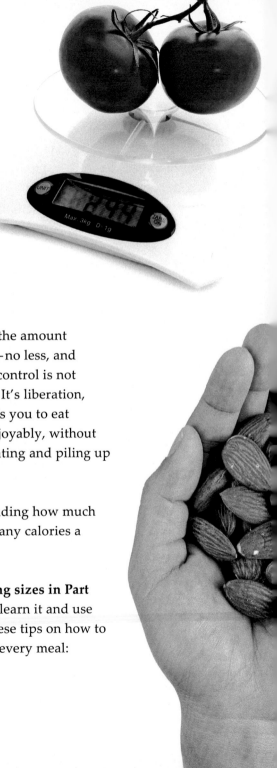

PORTION CONTROL: MAKE IT YOUR GOAL!

If you want to lose
weight, there's one thing
we'll state:
you gotta control what
you put on your plate!

This little ditty
expresses one of the
Rice Diet's fundamental
points: controlling how
much you eat is 100%
necessary to lose weight.
It's called portion control,
and it simply means eating the amount
of food that's right for you—no less, and
certainly, no more. Portion control is not
punishment or deprivation. It's liberation,
because portion control frees you to eat
sensibly, healthfully and enjoyably, without
risking the danger of overeating and piling up
excess calories.

Portion control is understanding how much
a serving size is and how many calories a
serving size contains.

**You'll find a guide to serving sizes in Part
Two of this book.** Study it, learn it and use
it. And as you do, follow these tips on how to
maintain portion control at every meal:

Plan your meals and snacks—Impulse eating—throwing stuff together from the fridge and pantry—is a recipe for overeating. Planning your meals and snacks makes you to think more about what you're eating, and how much you should eat.

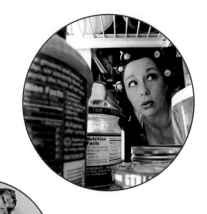

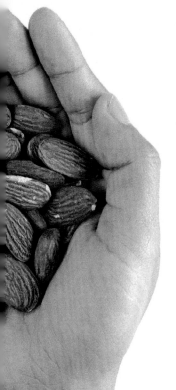

Proportion your portion—Divide your plate into quarter sections. One-half of your plate should contain an assortment of vegetables, preferably of different color, texture and taste. One-quarter of your plate should contain low-fat proteins, baked, broiled or grilled. And one-quarter of your plate should contain whole-grain starches.

Use smaller plates and glasses—When you eat and drink off smaller plates and glasses, you still feel like you're having your "regular" meal. It's amazing how this works, but it does; your stomach won't know the difference!

Start with a small serving—Instead of filling your plate with a full serving, fill it with half a serving. Eat slowly, put your knife and fork down often, and drink water. When you've finished your first half-serving, proceed to your second, and let it be your "seconds." It's a nice little trick that lets you have two helpings without eating "two" much.

Keep serving dishes off the table—Serve and eat your meal on individual plates, and keep serving dishes out of immediate reach. This will reduce the temptation to reach for seconds. And thirds. And...you get the idea.

Don't eat out of bags—Instead, open the bag, take out a small portion—and put the bag away! You won't miss what you can't see.

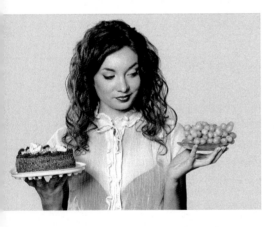

MAY YOU EAT SMART, LIVE LONG AND PROSPER

As you can see, eating sensibly is a simple concept, and the how-to rules and tips are easy to grasp. What's difficult is actually doing it. But remember, the bad eating habits you got into are just that—habits. You got into 'em, you can get out of 'em. And with some effort and willingness, eating sensibly can eventually be your habit. You'll be so much healthier and happier when you're eating the right foods in the right amounts. You'll feel so much better, and so much better about yourself. You'll enjoy life more, and for the first time in a long time, you'll get real satisfaction and enjoyment from the food you eat. Now all this...is food for thought.

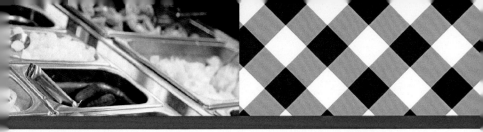

WHEN EATING OUT...

• **Think before you order**—Many meals in restaurants today are two to four times larger than you need, so make a plan before you order. Look for the menu online before you get to the restaurant, so you can plan what you'll order.

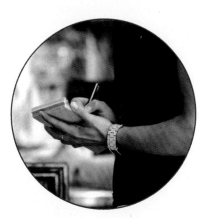

• **Eat half, take half home**— Order a to-go box before eating. Ask your server to put half your meal in a to-go box in the kitchen or to bring a to-go box to your table with your meal. You get portion control, and two meals for the price of one.

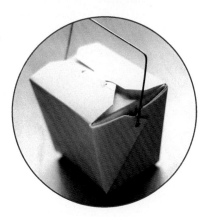

• **Smaller is better**—Order the smallest size of the food you want. If you can divide a bigger meal, and take half home for a second meal, go for it.

Refer to Chapter 8 for more information on eating out.

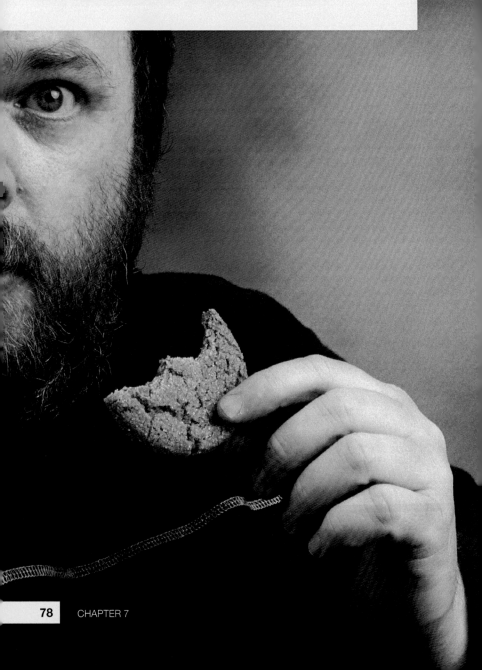

CHAPTER SEVEN
STRESS AND OVEREATING

"For fast-acting relief, try slowing down."
—Lily Tomlin

YOU KNOW STRESS ISN'T GOOD FOR YOUR HEALTH. You know there's a connection between stress and overeating. And yet, it's almost certain that stress and negative emotions continue to plague you, causing you to eat unhealthily, and diminishing the overall quality of your life. Of course, there will always be some stress and tension in our lives, that's just part of the human experience. And there are times when a certain level of stress can actually benefit us, by motivating us to successfully meet a challenge.

A simple example of this would be a student whose concern about failing a class motivates her to study and pass the final exam. In this case, a certain level of stress (concern about failing) caused her to take an appropriate action (studying) that led to a positive result (passing the exam).

In the case of overweight and obese people however, eating too much is sometimes the action taken to resolve stress. Clearly, this is not a good or effective solution; in fact, overeating only multiplies the problem, since it chains the eater to a vicious cycle of stress/eat/stress/eat/stress/eat. Eating doesn't resolve stress, and shortly after the feel-good meal or snack is eaten, the harmful emotions surface again.

See Chapter 17 for "The Cycle of Emotional Eating."

So what needs to be done? Simply put, we need to find ways to manage stress, to keep it at appropriate levels, like our studious student did, while preventing it from overwhelming and harming us. Yes, this is easier said than done. However, as with everything else about the Rice Diet, managing stress is not impossible. With the right understanding, and the use of stress management techniques, we can gain some control over our anxieties—instead of them controlling us.

START AT THE BEGINNING

With the knowledge that each of us is unique, we therefore possess different tolerances for stress, and different capabilities for dealing with it. Some people seem to be immune to anxiety, and nothing seems to rattle them; while others appear tightly wound and constantly on edge. And of course, there's a vast middle ground.

The starting point for managing your stress is to understand where you fall in these categories. Are you by nature an anxious person? Do you know which situations and occurrences cause you the greatest anxiety? Do you understand why these situations cause you such emotional turmoil? These are some of the questions you should ask and answer if you want to overcome overstress. We strongly suggest partnering with your doctor, religious leader, counselor or therapist in this quest for self-understanding. Your Rice Diet journal will also give you valuable insights into your emotional states and how you handle them, so please, fill in your journal every day.

STRESS MANAGEMENT: TRY THIS ....

There are many, many sources of information on the subject of stress management, which you can find at your local library, in bookstores, on the Internet, and certainly, through your doctor, religious leader or therapist. Take advantage of this information so easily at hand; a little reading and instruction on this subject can assist you tremendously in understanding your unique situation, and

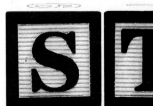
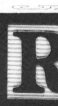

how to manage it. To get you started though, we offer the following stress reduction and management tips that you can practice immediately:

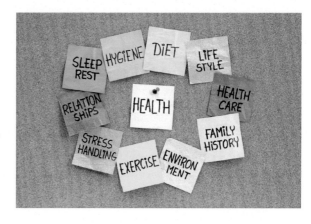

Get your stressful emotions out—
Keeping anger, frustration, sadness and other negative emotions inside you is like trying to cork the molten lava in a volcano. Releasing and expressing your emotions in an appropriate way is healthful on many levels, and there are many ways to do this, including:

- Expressing your feelings in your Rice Diet journal
- Talking with other Rice Dieters, or good listeners such as friends, family and counselors
- Expressing your feelings in art, be it poetry, music or drawing
- Expressing your feelings through crying (it's an excellent emotional release)

Cross food off your "answer" list—Make a list of things you can do to cope with stress—and include "EATING" on that list. Now, draw a big red line through that word, to remind yourself that of the many ways you can cope with stress, eating is definitely not one of them!

Know the signs of emotional hunger—We went over this in the last chapter, but it's worth repeating: normally, you should not be physically hungry until 4 to 6 hours after your previous meal. A growling stomach is a sign of physical hunger. If you're hungry shortly after a meal, or you don't detect

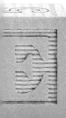
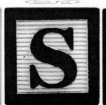
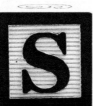

a physical sign of hunger, you're probably experiencing emotional (or "phantom") hunger; that is, the desire for food to appease your emotions. Feed your stomach only!

Get some exercise—We've said it before, and we'll say it again here: physical exercise has a wonderfully beneficial effect on one's emotional state. Medically speaking, exercise causes the release of certain neurotransmitters and hormones that alleviate emotional pain, elevate mood and increase energy. Physical exercise is Nature's anti-depressant, so when you get the blues, put on your walking shoes and you'll feel better.

Breathe deeply—Deep breathing is an age-old calming and anti-stress technique that you can do anywhere, anytime for relaxation.

Deep Breathing Exercises:
Sit up straight (do not arch your back). First exhale completely through your mouth. Place your hands on your stomach, just above your waist. Breathe in slowly through your nose, pushing your hands out with your stomach. This ensures that you are breathing deeply. Imagine that you are filling your body with air from the bottom up. *Hold* your breath to a count of two to five, or whatever you can handle. It is easier to hold your breath if you continue to hold out your stomach. Slowly and steadily breathe out through your mouth, feeling your hands move back in as you slowly contract your stomach, until most of the air is out. Exhalation is a little longer than inhalation. *You* can also do the above breathing exercise lying on your back. Deep breathing exercises can help you to relax before you go to sleep for the night, or fall back asleep if you awaken in the middle of the night. You can also practice deep breathing exercises standing – e.g. while sitting in traffic, or standing in a lineup at the grocery store. If you are really tense and feel as if you are holding your breath, simply concentrate on slowly breathing in and out.

Don't be a boredom binger—
Simple boredom or inactivity can also trigger the urge to overeat. The solution is to get busy with something besides going to the fridge or pantry. Make a list of your top 10 favorite activities and do one. Or make a list of chores that need to be done and take care of them. You'll feel a lot better doing something constructive instead of adding to your weight problem.

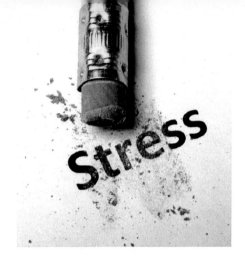

WE CAN'T STRESS THIS ENOUGH

Emotional eating caused by stress is one of the biggest contributors to weight problems and obesity. Successfully addressing this issue can go a long way toward helping you lose weight and regain your health. Everyone experiences stress from time to time, but people who learn to appropriately manage it are healthier and happier.

Exploring and confronting the root causes of our emotional turmoil requires honesty, courage and effort. Along the way, we may discover things about ourselves that are less than flattering; things about our behavior, attitude and actions that require change. We must abandon some of the old and truly harmful ways we've dealt with our emotions in favor of new and beneficial ones. Above all, we must realize that food does not solve, and never will solve, our emotional issues. Only we can do that. The good news—make that great news—is that it is possible to change. Thousands and thousands of successful Rice Dieters are proof of this, because the fact is, the Rice Diet can take the weight off everywhere. Including the weight on your shoulders.

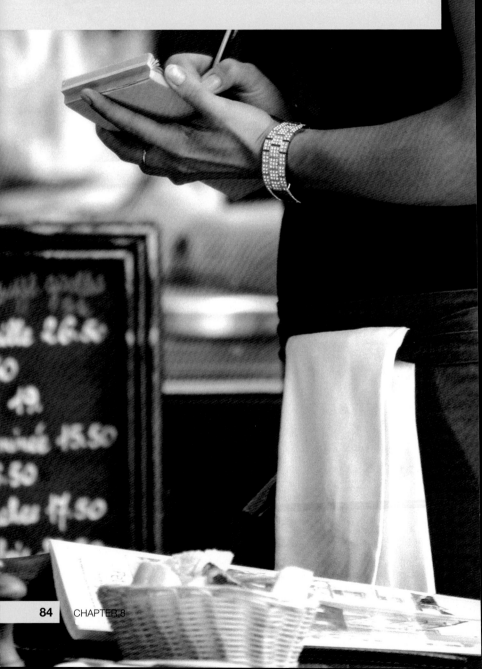

CHAPTER EIGHT
EATING RIGHT WHEN EATING OUT

"You can get anything you want at Alice's Restaurant..."
—Arlo Guthrie

IN OUR MOBILE, ON-THE-GO SOCIETY, EATING OUT IS MORE THAN AN OCCASIONAL ACTIVITY. These days, a lot of people eat at restaurants as often as they eat at home. After all, who doesn't like to put away the pots and pans and let someone else do the cooking, serving and cleaning up? As a Ricer, you too can enjoy meals out, but you need to be smart about it if you want to have your food and your weight loss, too.

Generally speaking, we recommend that you stay on the Rice Diet for 3 to 4 weeks before going out to a restaurant. This gives you time to adjust to the diet and its requirements, and practice some of the eating and self-control techniques. We realize, though, that this may not be possible, especially if you travel frequently. No matter whether you've been on the diet for a day or a year, there are guidelines for eating out the Rice Diet way. Let's look at them.

CHOOSE YOUR RESTAURANT WISELY

Most commercial establishments do not prepare food in a manner consistent with the Rice Diet. Commercially prepared foods are generally high in sodium, fat and sugar, and are often fried or drenched in sauces. Even meals labeled as "healthy choice" and the like may be light in calories and fat, but still contain heavy amounts of sodium. You must avoid these traps, and you can do so by:

• Previewing the restaurant's menu online
• Calling ahead to make the establishment aware of your health concerns, and confirming that it will prepare your meal according to your Rice Diet specifications. Reconfirm this upon arrival.

• Requesting how you want your meal prepared; a good restaurant easily can and will do this. And if the establishment can't comply with your requests—choose another.

ON THE MENU: THINGS TO AVOID, THINGS TO CHOOSE

As a Ricer eating out, your goal should be to enjoy a delicious, satisfying and filling meal that conforms to your diet. You can do this by avoiding some things and choosing others.

AVOID	CHOOSE
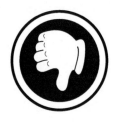	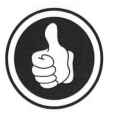

AVOID

• Fried, sautéed, stuffed or breaded foods
• Bread and crackers (bring your own Rice Diet-recommended ones)
• Butter and buttered dishes
• Pickles and relish
• Croutons, Parmesan cheese, bacon bits and raisins
• ALL dressings that are not low-calorie, low-sodium and non-fat
• Sliced or chopped whole eggs
• High-sodium food preparations (ask your server to have the Chef prepare food without salt)
• ALL sauces and creams

CHOOSE

• Broiled, grilled, poached or boiled dishes. Any dish that can be fried, sautéed, stuffed or breaded can be cooked in these four ways instead.
• Steamed or grilled vegetables
• Non-fat, low-calorie, low-sodium dressings such as balsamic vinaigrette (or bring your own)
• Cucumbers, tomatoes, sliced green peppers and lettuce
• Pineapple chunks
• Fresh fruits for dessert

AT THE START OF YOUR MEAL

First, don't go into a restaurant famished: that's just a temptation to indulge in bread or rolls. Have a light snack and drink water shortly before you go out. When you arrive at your table, you'll probably be offered a bread basket in short order. Decline it, and ask if they serve low-calorie, low fat, unsalted crackers instead (2-3 crackers make a serving; bring your own if necessary). Before your meal

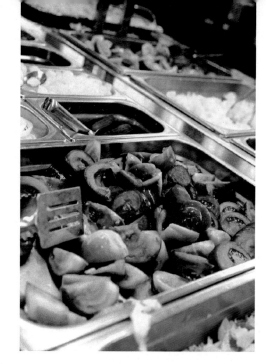

arrives, drink a glass of water; it's a healthy appetite suppressant and prepares your digestive system for the meal to come.

Also, before you begin your meal, enlist the cooperation of your server by indicating you have health concerns and would appreciate their accommodating your dietary requirements.

SALADS AND SALAD BARS

These obviously are good choices, so long as you select the right ingredients and dressings. When you order a salad or the salad bar, make sure you only use a non-fat, low-sodium, low-calorie dressing, such as balsamic vinaigrette. And don't pour salad dressing on your salad. Instead, ask for it on the side and dip your fork into it lightly before you take a bite of salad. That way you'll use the minimum amount of dressing but still taste the flavors. Croutons, nuts, cheese and seeds should also be avoided; ask for extra vegetables in their place.

HAVE YOUR ENTRÉE YOUR WAY

When your entrée comes, make sure it's the way you ordered it—the Ricer way. Are the steamed vegetables you ordered covered in butter or sauce? Was your chicken or fish grilled without seasoning or sauce as you requested? If any portion of your meal is not prepared as you ordered, tell your server to take it back and have it prepared the way you asked. Be polite but firm; you're the customer, and you're paying them good money to prepare the meal the way you want it.

Here are some other things to look at when your entrée arrives:

- Most restaurants heavily salt their rice. If you want rice, ask that it be low-sodium, and request that the server confirm it.
- Order a dry baked potato if you like, but request that the skin remain unsalted (many restaurants salt potato skins). If your potato skin is salted, just eat the inside and leave the skin untouched.
- Stay clear of garnishes, relishes and pickles, as they're loaded with salt.
- Don't drink sodas or soda water; even the diet options are heavy on sodium. Drink carbonated water instead.

FOR DESSERT

Don't let a sugar/fat/ sodium/calorie-laden dessert spoil your meal. Your desserts should only be fresh fruits, at least for the first few months of your diet. If there is a fruit you want, and you don't see it on the menu, ask your waiter anyway; you never know what he might be able to find in the kitchen. You should

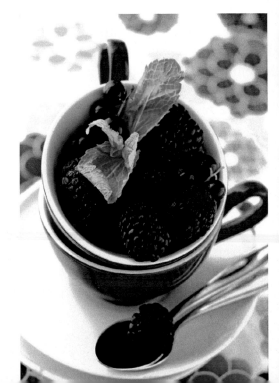

also avoid adding nuts or whipped cream to your fruit unless you've calculated the added calories and fats, and are permitted them.

REMEMBER YOUR PORTION CONTROL TIPS
In Chapter Six, you learned three good tips for controlling your meal portions when you eat out. They're worth repeating here.

Think before you order—Look for the menu online before you get to the restaurant, so you know what you'll order.

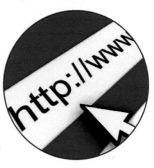

Eat half, take half home— Order a to-go box before eating. Have half of your meal put in a to-go box before you begin your meal, and take that portion home for a second meal.

Smaller is better—Order the smallest size of the food you want. If you can divide a bigger meal, and take half home for a second meal, go for it.

EATING OUT THE RICE WAY IS THE RIGHT WAY
Keeping to your Rice Diet and enjoying a nice meal out is pretty easy—provided you follow the rules. Yes, there are some things you can't eat and some types of preparation you must avoid, but why dwell on them? Think instead of all the good things you can eat. You're getting the best of both culinary worlds: a delicious, satisfying meal and a healthy one that meets your dietary needs. Looking at it that way, there's no reason to envy others who "eat whatever they want"—in fact, they may be the unfortunate ones, because they're filling up on food that isn't good for them.

When you eat out, a check isn't the only way you pay for what you've eaten. You also pay a price for eating wrong. That's something you won't have to worry about if you eat out the Rice Diet way.

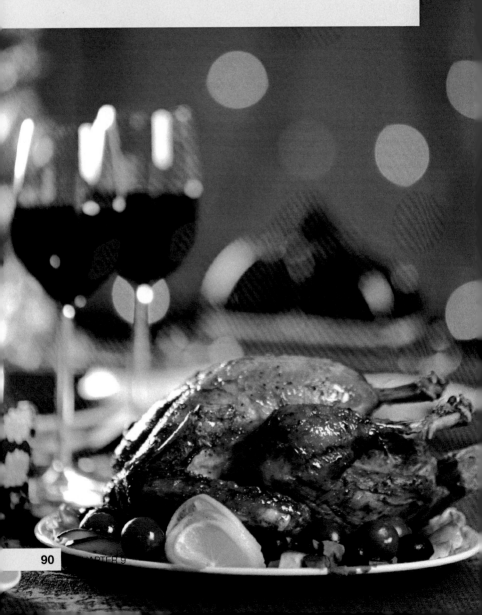

CHAPTER NINE
EATING DURING HOLIDAYS

> ## *"Gluttony and surfeiting are no proper occasions for thanksgiving."*
> —Charles Lamb

THANKSGIVING, Christmas and Chanukah, New Year's Eve, Easter, Memorial Day Weekend, the Fourth of July, Labor Day Weekend: the American calendar is filled with holidays that seem to provide excuses for filling ourselves with food. And who are we to be party poopers? Food, being the wonderful, glorious thing that it is, should be a part of any celebration or holiday. When we gather together with family and friends, sharing meals is about the most natural, celebratory activity we can imagine. As a Rice Dieter, you can join in the holiday fun by simply remembering this:

The holidays are a time to celebrate, and by sticking to your Rice Diet, you can celebrate losing weight, reversing your medical conditions, feeling and looking your best, and enjoying life to the fullest.

Now let's be honest: of all the challenges faced by a dedicated Ricer, maintaining your diet during the holidays is one of the biggest. But the eating tips and strategies we'll share in this chapter will give you tools to avoid unhealthy eating, stick to your diet—and quite possibly, enjoy your celebration more than ever.

The one thing we can't give you is commitment and dedication. That comes from you. Just being a Ricer says you're committed to losing weight and changing your life for the better. The holidays are a big test of your commitment, we understand. But if you take it one day at a time, and practice living the Rice Diet lifestyle each and every day, you can enjoy the taste of the sweetest thing yet: success!

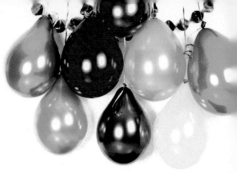

HOLIDAY HELPERS: HELPFUL SUGGESTIONS ON HEALTHY HOLIDAY EATING

The best way to stay with your Rice Diet over a holiday is through preparation, using the tips and suggestions below to eat sensibly and enjoy the holiday without slipping:

Plan ahead—If you're hosting a holiday gathering, decide what things you'll serve and be sure that healthy, Rice Diet foods and snacks are among then. If you're a guest, bring a dish or two of wholesome food for yourself and others to enjoy.

Turn to your Rice Diet journal—As part of your daily entries, make a list of holiday diet concerns you have, reflecting on:
- How you've handled holiday eating in the past (both failures and successes)
- How you wish to handle things differently
- The steps you'll take to stay with your diet during the holiday

Build your confidence with resolution reminders—Do these simple things to maintain your commitment to your diet and your health over holidays:
- Keep a "Before" photo of yourself handy to remind you of the consequences of back sliding
- Create a "Reasons to Lose Weight" list featuring the specific reasons why you'd like to lose weight. Keep it with you and review it daily.
- Memorize and recite affirmations (see index) that speak to your ability to be successful with your diet. Create your own special holiday affirmation, and make it your motto for healthy holiday eating.

Snack lightly before the party—You don't want to arrive at a holiday gathering totally famished. To avoid this, have a healthy snack and drink a glass or two of water before you hit the party. This will help prevent the urge to fill up on the wrong foods. Mushrooms and oatmeal are great appetite suppressors, so look for ways to incorporate them in your holiday diet.

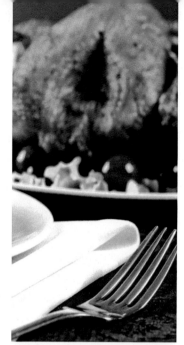

Be assertive, protect your health!— "Have some." "Try this." "Just a taste won't hurt you." You hear a lot of this over holidays, as people, for good or ill, try to tempt you off your regimen. Don't let other people dictate your food choices and your health! Instead, choose one of these polite yet firm responses:
• "No thanks, not right now."
• "No thanks, I'm really full."
• "No thanks, I'd really like some more (insert healthy food here) instead."
If someone tries to push some unhealthy food on you, push it away!

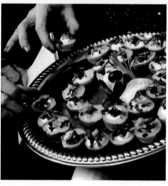

Ask yourself this—Before you indulge in diet-busting food, ask yourself, "How will I feel after eating this?" Knowing you've cheated on your diet is hardly likely to make you happy. What's more, if you've been on your Rice Diet awhile, you'll find that processed foods loaded with sodium, sugar and fat make you feel bad physically. So ask yourself, "Why in the heck would I want to feel lousy and spoil my holiday?"

Enjoy the company of supportive family and friends—Socialize with people who understand and encourage your decision to live a healthy lifestyle, especially other Rice Dieters. Choose the company of positive thinking people and avoid the naysayers.

Keep alcohol consumption to a minimum—Alcohol adds calories, plus it can cloud your judgment and weaken your will. Have a glass of water with a twist of lemon or lime, or fill your champagne glass with carbonated water instead.

Have fun without food—Try to engage in activities that are not food-related, such as playing board games, or walking with friends to view holiday displays or fireworks shows. Walking around your neighborhood beats grazing around the table, so get up and get out with some like-minded friends. And speaking of walking, here's a reminder: **DON'T TAKE A HOLIDAY FROM EXERCISING** during a holiday. Stay with your exercise program, and use the holiday time off to get in shape.

Don't gain. Instead, maintain—It's hard to lose weight over a holiday. But that's no excuse for gaining pounds. If you can't lose weight over a holiday, make it your goal to maintain your weight during the festivities, and then continue with your weight loss regimen after the holiday is over.

REMEMBER, HEALTHY HOLIDAYS ARE HAPPY HOLIDAYS

For some people, overeating and lack of exercise are holiday traditions. That's sad, especially considering that holidays are a time to celebrate life—and you can't enjoy a quality life without good health. If gorging on food and undermining your well-being has been part of your past holidays, compare that to the holidays you can enjoy by staying with your Rice Diet. Think of the energy and mental lift you get from exercising. Think how good it feels to be trimmer, healthier, happier; to be free of the medical problems caused by obesity. Think of the boost to your self-confidence, knowing that you can stay with your diet, face the holiday temptations—and prevail. When you compare these two scenarios, there really is no comparison. Healthy holidays are the way to go.

We hope this section of the book becomes dog-eared, as you refer to it from Thanksgiving through Labor Day. Read and reread our tips, commit to them and practice them. And have a very, very happy holiday!

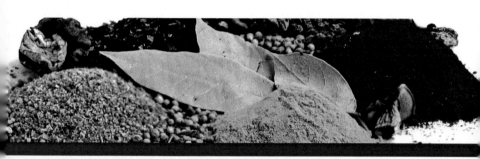

SPICE UP YOUR HOLIDAYS

Healthy eating and tasty eating go hand in hand when you add spices to your food. Try these spices in your holiday meals or any time of year:

Mrs. Dash (all varieties)

Basil	Oregano
Chili Pepper	Paprika
Cilantro	Parsley
Cinnamon	Pepper
Coriander	Rosemary
Cumin	Tarragon
Garlic	Thyme
Ginger	Turmeric
Mint	
Nutmeg	

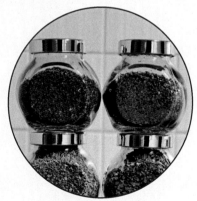

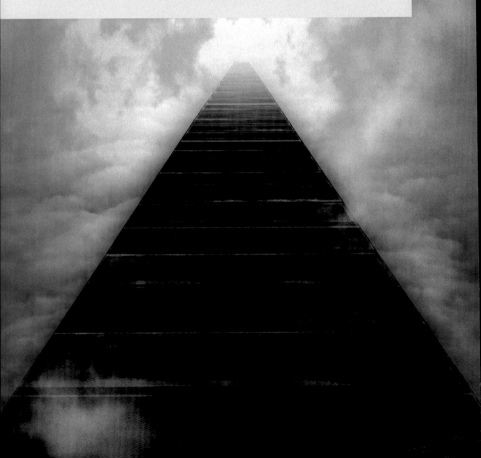

CHAPTER TEN
FEAR, FRUSTRATION, FOOD PUSHERS AND SABOTEURS

> ## *"A champion is someone who gets up, even when he can't."*
> ## —Jack Dempsey

MAINTAINING A DIET IS LIKE CLIMBING A MOUNTAIN: there's crowning glory at the top, and lots of rocks to get past in between. There are many obstacles to staying with your diet, some caused by yourself, and some by others (including even your best-intentioned but misguided friends and family members). Chances are, you'll come up against some of these obstacles—almost every Ricer does. But with a little knowledge, and the right coping strategies, you can overcome them—as all successful Ricers do. Let's look at some of the challenges we face, and how to deal with them.

FEAR OF FAILURE

Chances are, you've tried dieting before and haven't been successful. You may feel discouraged, and even embarrassed, especially if your weight has yo-yo'd up and down during your attempts. Under these circumstances, it's easy to think you can't succeed at dieting, and making another attempt will only result in further disappointment and humiliation. You've tried and tried, and you're afraid to try again.

But maybe…just maybe…your fears are not as real, or as forbidding, as you imagine. After all, you probably have at least a few examples in your own life of mastering something gradually after frustration and setbacks. If you play a musical instrument, you surely had some "I can't play this darn thing" moments before you got the hang of it. Or remember how intimidating it was the first few times you got behind the wheel of a car when you learned how to drive? Failure at first—or second or third—is a common experience to all people, but not all failures are final.

If you still insist on beating yourself up for your lack of success, consider this: some of history's most successful people ...were failures:

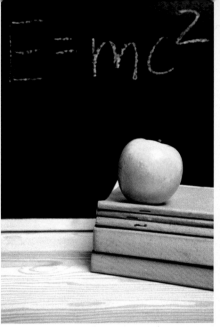

- Albert Einstein was expelled from school and refused admittance into the Zurich Polytechnic School
- Ludwig van Beethoven was considered by one of his music teachers to be "completely hopeless as a composer"
- Henry Ford failed and went broke five times before he succeeded
- Michael Jordan was cut from his high school basketball team
- Author Jack London received 600 rejection slips before he sold his first story

These folks all had three things in common: 1) they failed 2) they persisted, and 3) they ultimately succeeded. Sure they were bright and talented, but that wasn't what got them past failure. It was PERSISTENCE, the simple refusal to abandon their dream and give up. We can all relate to this. When it comes to fear of failure, take to heart the immortal words of President Franklin D. Roosevelt: "We have nothing to fear but fear itself."

THE WEIGHT LOSS PLATEAU

After starting your Rice Diet, you may lose a fair amount of weight rather quickly. But after a while, the pounds seem to come off more slowly, or hardly at all. You have now arrived at a weight loss plateau, a stage where you lose almost no additional weight despite continued dieting and exercise. What causes a weight plateau? According to MayoClinic.com:

A plateau occurs because your metabolism—the process of burning calories for energy—slows as you lose lean tissue (muscle). When you lose weight, you lose both fat and lean tissue. (The notion that overweight people have a slower metabolism is a myth. In general, the higher a person's weight, the higher the body's metabolic rate.) Your weight-loss efforts result in a new equilibrium with your now slower metabolism. This means that in order to lose more weight, you need to increase activity or decrease the calories you eat. Using the same approach that worked initially will maintain your weight loss, but it won't lead to more weight loss.

Reaching a weight loss plateau is normal, but it can also be very discouraging, especially after the noticeable success you've initially experienced. You believe you've gone as far as you can go on your diet, you slacken up on your program, and more often than not, the calories and your weight begin to creep back up.

The truth is, a weight loss plateau doesn't indicate you've reached the limits of your diet. Rather, it indicates that some changes to your regimen are necessary. Here are some of the things you can do:

Review your program— Have you increased your calorie consumption or slacked off on your exercising? Review your Rice Diet journal to make sure you're on track with your regimen. You may also want to consult your doctor for advice.

Exercise more—Additional exercise will cause you to burn more calories, so look for ways to increase the length and intensity of your daily exercises.

Become more active—Simply increasing your daily physical activity can help you lose additional weight. Gardening, house cleaning and walking instead of driving are just some of the things you can do to pick up the pace of your activity.

A weight loss plateau should not derail your Rice Diet. Just remember that it's normal, and by taking the right steps, you can move past it.

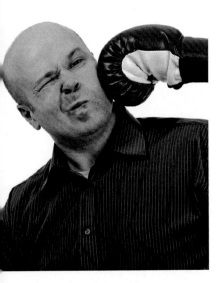

DON'T LET SABOTEURS AND FOOD PUSHERS PUSH YOU!

Whether they're just trying to be nice, or trying to set you up for failure, people who try to sabotage your diet or push bad food on you are jeopardizing your good health. No one should be permitted to do that. It can be hard to resist saboteurs and food pushers, especially if they are friends or family members who mean well and believe that deviating from or abandoning your diet won't hurt you. But as a Ricer, you know better.

SABOTEURS AND FOOD PUSHERS: WHO ARE THEY?

Anyone who tries to get you off your diet (either deliberately or though ignorance of your condition) is a saboteur or food pusher. Their motivations may differ, but their actions can lead to the same bad result: compromising your diet and health. To effectively handle saboteurs and food pushers, you must first be able to recognize them. Here are some indicators:

Saboteurs—
- May make negative or snide remarks about your diet and your commitment to it
- Will try to get you to eat your old favorite foods
- Can be motivated by insecurity, resentment or fear of your success with your diet
- Can also be motivated by good intentions based on ignorance of your health requirements

Food pushers—
- May use subterfuge to persuade you to get off your diet. Example: "You look great just the way you are!"
- May try to "force" unhealthy foods on you when you have not asked for them
- May try to tempt you into getting off your diet by asking you if you want something they know is not good for you
- Can be motivated by ignorance of your health requirements or a desire to prevent your success with your diet

Some saboteurs and food pushers may intentionally try to derail your diet for their own (unfortunately) perverse reasons. But many of these people act with what they believe are the best intentions, encouraging you to "enjoy life" a little more by eating the very foods that caused your problems. Whether ill- or well-intentioned, any appeals to compromise or quit your diet must be resisted–in the interest of your good health!

RESPONDING TO SABOTEURS AND FOOD PUSHERS

It's not always easy fending off someone who is determined to wreck your diet. But it must be done, and it's your responsibility to do it. Whenever you're pushed, a polite but firm refusal to budge is the only answer. Here are some good responses to saboteur and food pusher invitations:

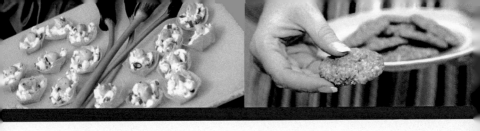

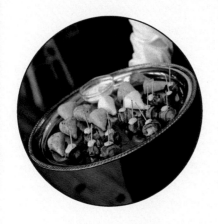

FOOD PUSHER SCENARIOS

Food Pusher: Have another slice of pie! Blueberry is your favorite!
You: Thanks, but do you think I could take a slice home instead for later?

Food Pusher: You kidding? One piece, one bite, it can't hurt.
You: I really can't eat another bite, I'm so full now. It was so good I don't want to feel sick afterwards.

Food Pusher: Are you a rabbit, do you just eat salads?
You: It might seem that way, but no, I love salads and enjoy eating them. Besides, it works for me!

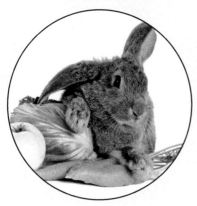

Food Pusher: Wow, the rest of the family doesn't eat like you do, so what's up with the diet?
You: The rest of the family eats food that they enjoy and that's great for them, but it doesn't work for me, and I can't compare myself to them.

Food Pusher: Is that all you think about, your calories? What a drag, you gotta have more fun.
You: Yeah, I know it may seem like that and you seemed concerned, thanks, but I'm happy to keep track of what I'm eating, it makes me feel good.

In a pinch, remember, a polite "no, thank you" communicates your wishes quite clearly. If a saboteur or food pusher becomes persistent, just tell the person you're losing weight for your health, on your doctor's orders. That way, it's your doctor who's "refusing" the food, all in the interest of your well-being. Knowing that some saboteurs and food pushers offer food out of misguided kindness, be sure to compliment them on the good foods they serve, such as garden salads, fresh fruit and the like. This sends a clear message as to what food you enjoy and prefer.

As we've said before, the Rice Diet is a diet in name only. In reality, it's a healthy lifestyle choice that anyone who truly cares about you will encourage and support. Perhaps the best strategy for dealing with saboteurs and food pushers is to simply say, "I'm committed to a healthy lifestyle and there are some foods I've dropped from my diet. But I'm not complaining—I feel better than ever!"

LAST BUT NOT LEAST: SLIP-UPS

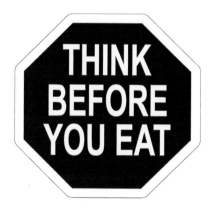

Committing to your diet 50% or 80% just won't work. You need total commitment. That said, no one is perfect, and we all stumble from time to time. It's how we handle our slip-ups and setbacks that matter. We can turn them into little blips on the path of progress, regrettable but nothing more. Or we can let them snowball into…well, an avalanche that wrecks our diet and our dreams. But we don't want that, do we? Good. So let's look at what to do should we fall off our diet.

The first thing you should do if you slip-up is to forgive yourself — without excusing yourself. Your slip-up is a simple acknowledgement of what every dieter knows all too well: dieting is not easy. You're neither the first nor the last person to go astray on a diet. At the same time, you need to take responsibility for your action, instead of trying to deflect it with excuses and rationalizations. Try saying this to yourself:

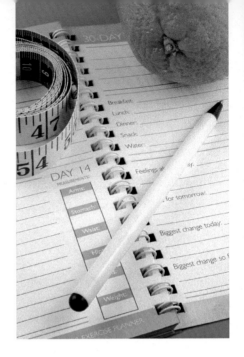

"I'm responsible for my health, and I've done something to compromise my good health. I take responsibility for my actions, and I take responsibility for correcting them, in the interest of my happiness and well-being. I'm a responsible person, and this is an opportunity to prove that. I am grateful for this opportunity."

Now that you've taken responsibility, and turned your slip-up into an opportunity for growth and improvement, the next step is to:

GET RIGHT BACK ON YOUR RICE DIET. DO IT THE VERY NEXT MEAL AFTER YOUR SLIP-UP!

The less time between your slip-up and resuming your Rice Diet lifestyle, the better — and the easier for you. Getting back on your diet immediately means less disruption of your healthy routine, and you won't lose time to guilt, hand-wringing and other fruitless behavior either.

While we hardly recommend dwelling on your setbacks, we strongly recommend that you write about them in your journal — not to beat up on yourself, but to learn from your experience. Briefly, what was the nature of your slip-up? What do you believe triggered the event? What steps do you plan to take to avoid this problem in the future? Pondering and answering these questions in your Rice Diet journal can lead to amazing epiphanies that give you insights into your challenges and how to solve them. Along with journaling, seek the support and counsel of other Ricers, or people in your support network. They know what you're going through because they've been there themselves, and they can help you get past your difficulties.

"THE WINNER AND STILL CHAMPION IS ..."

In boxing champion Jack Dempsey's world, the winner of the fight was the man left standing. While dieting isn't exactly a heavyweight prizefight (thank goodness!), it too requires tenacity, courage and determination. Just remember, when you encounter obstacles on the road to good health, you can choose to overcome them, and turn them into positive experiences that make you stronger and more confident in your ability to succeed. Like a boxer, you may experience some knockdowns—but that doesn't mean your down for the count.

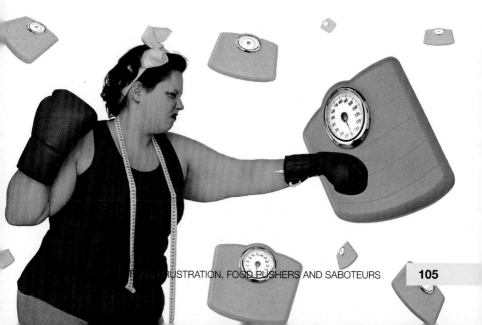

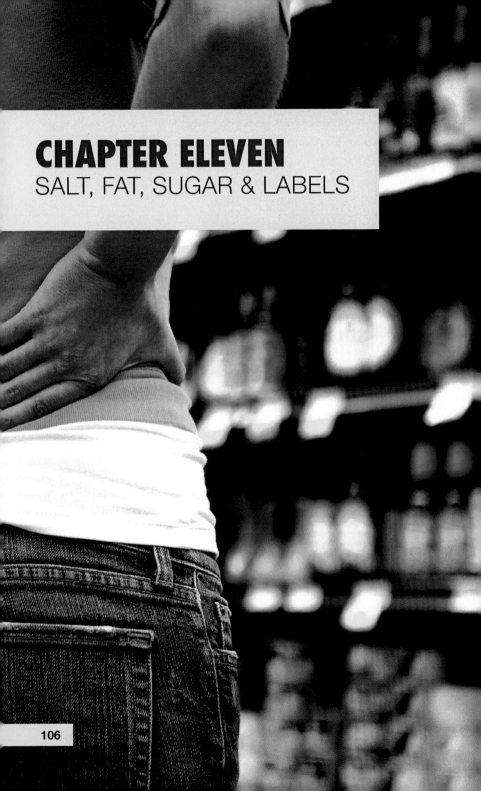

CHAPTER ELEVEN
SALT, FAT, SUGAR & LABELS

"There is no end of craving. Hence contentment alone is the best way to happiness."
—Sivananda

JUST ABOUT EVERYONE LOVES SALT, FAT AND SUGAR. But virtually none of us needs all the salt, fat and sugar you'll find in much of today's popular foods. To appease our cravings (and make lots of money, too), many food manufacturers have loaded their products with frightening amounts of these additives. The result is food at its worst: harmful, unhealthy and addicting. As a Ricer, you'll want to zealously regulate your intake of the Big Bad Three to ensure you're not getting more than is necessary for your health. Doing this requires a little planning and oversight—and a little more discipline and self-control. You'll find though, that once you've cut your intake of salt, fat and sugar, your body quickly adjusts to their absence. In fact, you'll come to feel much better without these additives in your system. It's a matter of weaning yourself off them, then feeding your body more healthy alternatives. We'll discuss this in a moment, but first, let's look at the three big offenders of the American diet:

SALT

Salt is composed of two chemicals, sodium and chloride. Each one has important uses in the body: sodium helps maintain normal blood pressure and normal function of muscles and nerves while chloride helps keep your body fluids in proper balance. Salt is essential for good health, at least in small amounts, but too much salt can raise blood pressure, leading to hypertension, strokes and other serious medical problems. The risk of elevated blood pressure increases with age, so it is increasingly important to regulate your salt intake as you advance in years.

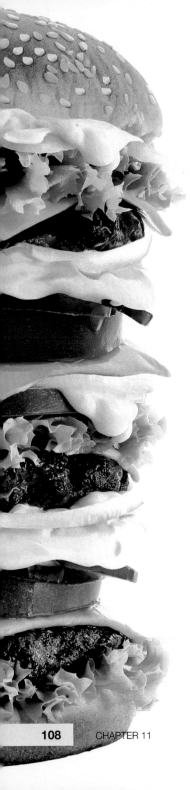

FAT

From ice cream to burgers, foods cooked in fat, or with fat added, have a texture, smell and taste that seems almost irresistible (although this is merely learned behavior that can also be unlearned). It's true that fat gives you energy, and a certain amount of it can be beneficial to your health. The problem is, fat contains lots of energy, and if we don't burn it all off (through vigorous exercise, for example), our bodies simply store up the fat, and that can make us—well, fat. It helps if you stick to healthy fats, such as those contained in sunflower oil and olive oil, and avoid unhealthy ones, such as hydrogenated fats and saturated fats found in butter, lard, meats and cheeses. These unhealthy fats, also called hard fats, can clog your arteries and restrict your blood flow, leading to heart disease.

SUGAR

Sugar is a heavenly taste sensation, plus it provides needed energy for your body. So what's wrong with that? Well, this: sugar is in just about everything you eat, including the good stuff like fruits, so it's very easy to get more—much more—than is good for you.

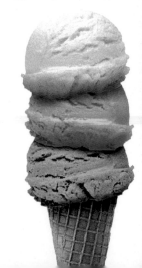

And when your body has more sugar than it needs, it converts that sugar into…fat. What's more, sugar contains no proteins, minerals or vitamins. It's all about energy and fat. Naturally, you'll need to watch the amount of sugar you consume daily, but in addition to that, you'll want to:

• Avoid refined white sugar or high-fructose corn syrup, which are the sweetening staples of much processed foods and soda
• Get your sugar from fruits, raw honey, molasses and other natural sources

AVOID THE SNACK ATTACK
Quick tips to stay on track and avoid the snack attack:

• During holidays such as Halloween, don't buy candy that you like and you won't be tempted to eat it.

• Purchase snack size packages of candies, maybe gummies, ones that you could even help yourself to occasionally and not get into too much trouble.

• Don't fool yourself into thinking those containing nuts or fruit are nutritious or otherwise good for you. Candy is candy and shouldn't be part of your regimen.

• If you do have an occasional sweet tooth, seek out sugar free candies: Brach's makes a large assortment of sugar free candy which won't get you into too much trouble if you are able to practice portion control.

• Keep track: This one sounds funny but keeping the candy wrappers in front of you will remind you how many you have eaten.

• Have a huge bowl of fruit visible on the table or sideboard. When you are craving a sweet, reach for a piece of fruit.

• Chewing sugar free minty gum will always create a clean fresh feeling in your mouth, keeping you from wanting to chew on candy instead.

SPICE THINGS UP

If you want to kick the salt habit and still add some tasty kick to your food, try these spices and herbs. The different flavors they add, alone or in combination, can turn the most basic dish into something special. Try them all, get creative, and bon appétit!

- Allspice, ground
- Anise seed
- Basil
- Bay leaf
- Caraway seed
- Celery seed
- Chili powder
- Cinnamon, ground
- Cloves, ground
- Coriander seed
- Cumin seed
- Curry powder
- Dill weed
- Fennel seed
- Garlic powder
- Ginger, ground
- Mace, ground
- Marjoram
- MSG
- Mustard seed
- Nutmeg, ground
- Onion powder
- Oregano
- Paprika
- Parsley
- Pepper, black
- Pepper, cayenne
- Pepper, white
- Rosemary
- Sage
- Saffron
- Salt
- Tarragon
- Thyme
- Turmeric, ground
- Vanilla extract
- Vinegar

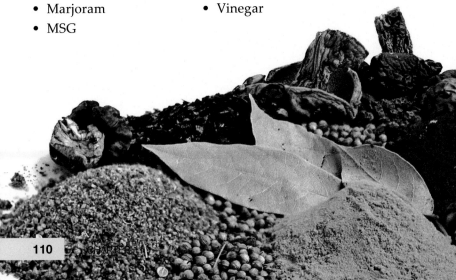

READ THE LABELS

Reading food labels when you shop is one of the best ways to measure your intake of salt, fat, sugar and other ingredients. Here are some guidelines to help you better understand the claims on food labels.

- *Low calorie*: 40 calories or less per serving
- *Fat free*: Less than 0.5g of saturated fat per serving
- *Saturated fat free*: Less than 0.5g of saturated fat and less than 0.5g of trans fatty acids
- *Low saturated fat*: 1g or less of saturated fat per serving
- *Low sodium*: 140mg of sodium or less per serving
- *Very low sodium*: 35mg of sodium or less per serving
- *Sodium free (or salt free)*: Less than 5mg of sodium per serving
- *Reduced sodium*: At least 25 percent less sodium per serving than the regular version
- *Cholesterol free*: Less than 2mg of cholesterol per serving
- *Low cholesterol*: 20mg or less of cholesterol per serving
- *Reduced cholesterol*: At least 25 percent less cholesterol per serving than the regular version
- *Sugar free*: Less than 500mg of sugar per serving
- *Reduced sugar*: At least 25 percent less sugar per serving than the regular version
- *High fiber*: 5g or more of fiber per serving
- *Good source of fiber*: 2.5 to 4.9g of fiber per serving
- *Serving size*: The serving size is listed at the top of the label. While a food item may appear low in fat or calories, you might notice the serving size is tiny. Keep this in mind when measuring portions.
- *Calories*: Calories provide a measurement of how much energy you obtain after eating a serving size of a specific food.
- *Nutrients*: The nutrients listed on a food label refer to total fat, saturated fat, cholesterol, carbohydrates (including fiber and added sugars), protein, vitamins A and C, calcium and iron. Other nutrients may be included at the manufacturer's discretion.

- *Percent daily values*: These listings provide an estimate of the percentage of a nutrient from one serving in a typical 2000-calorie diet:
  - If a food provides 5 percent or less of a nutrient, it is considered a poor source of that nutrient.
  - Food that provides 10 to 20 percent of your daily recommended amount of a nutrient is a good source of that nutrient.
  - If a food provides more than 20 percent of a nutrient, it is considered high in that nutrient.
- *Ingredient list*: The ingredient list is always ordered from the most prominent ingredient to the least. Beware of foods that list sugar (including high fructose corn syrup or sucrose), fats, oils or salt as one of their first two ingredients. These are not your healthiest choices.

THE MORE YOU KNOW, THE BETTER YOU EAT

Knowing what's in your food is essential to the success of your diet. It's tempting to indulge in things loaded with salt, fat and sugar, but just remember, you pay a very high price for these indulgences when you allow these health-damaging substances into your body. And keep this in mind, too: there are many delicious and filling alternatives to the Big Bad Three, including a host of spices, herbs and oils, that you can eat without harm—or guilt! And yes, we know it takes some patience and vigilance to read the labels before you buy the food, but just because a package has big splashy words like "All Natural!" or "Made With Real Fruit!" doesn't mean you can pluck it off the shelf without examining the contents. Read the labels to determine whether or not the item belongs in your diet. Always choose the right foods over the wrong ones. After all, it's your health—and your money— that keeps food companies in business, so don't squander your well-being or your cash on food that doesn't belong in your Rice Diet lifestyle.

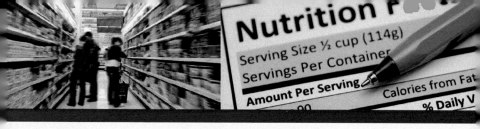

TWO LABELS. WHAT'S THE DIFFERENCE?

Here are nutrition labels for two different sauces. Each serving size is 1/2 cup. Which has more calories and fat? Which has more sodium?

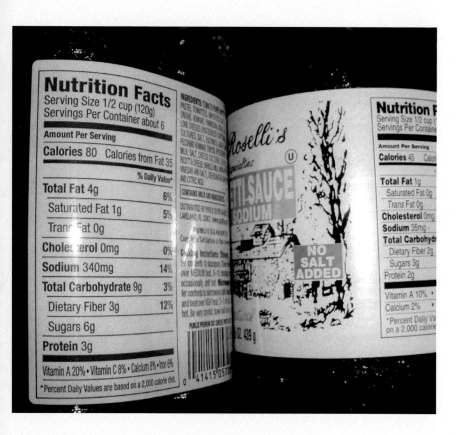

CHAPTER TWELVE
MAINTAINING YOUR WEIGHT LOSS

> *"The difference between try and triumph is just a little umph."*
> —Marvin Phillips

LOSING 100% OF YOUR EXCESS WEIGHT…is half the battle. The other half, of course, is keeping the weight off for good. This can be a challenge, but as Rice Diet creator Dr. Walter Kempner observed, if you are able to maintain your ideal body weight for two years, you should be able to maintain it for the rest of your life. As countless Ricers have proved, this is DOABLE so long as you stick to your Rice Diet regimen of proper eating, exercise, motivation and a little self-discipline. Here are some tips to help you keep off the weight you've worked so hard to lose:

Weigh yourself daily—This is the simplest, easiest way to make sure you're maintaining your ideal weight. The scales don't lie, and if you see the numbers creeping up you know you must take immediate corrective action.

Go back to Week 1—If you gain 3-5 pounds, immediately go back to Week 1 of your Rice Diet regimen until you have lost this excess weight. This type of weight gain can usually be attributed to excessive sodium ingestion, and losing the weight should only take 2-7 days.

Continue your exercise regimen—Keep it up at least 5 days a week. Exercise is the best way to burn calories, and burning calories helps keep the weight off.

Make your eating structured and simple—Stick to a basic, repetitious eating regimen and only allow yourself 1-2 days a week to eat a bit more liberally.

Be mindful of your medical requirements—If you are hypertensive, keep your sodium intake to under 1000 mg per day. If you are diabetic, avoid all refined sugars that are added to commercial foods. If you have heart disease or high lipid levels, keep your fat intake down to 10%-20% of your daily calories (usually between 30-35g per day).

Continue to monitor the foods in your home—Don't let the bad ones "sneak" back into your kitchen or pantry! If they aren't there, you won't be tempted to eat them, and you'll greatly decrease your chances of cheating.

WATCH YOUR DAILY CALORIC INTAKE—DAILY!

Keeping a daily track of the calories you consume is a good idea when you're losing weight and for maintaining your ideal weight. The number of calories you can consume daily on the Rice Diet depends on your age, metabolism, activity level, current weight and goal weight. Here is how to calculate your basal metabolic rate (BMR), which will give you your targeted calorie intake to maintain your weight:

Step 1

Harris Benedict Formula for Women

BMR = 655 + (9.6 X weight in kilos) + (1.8 X height in cm) - (4.7 X age in years).

Harris Benedict Formula for Men

BMR = 66 + (13.7 X weight in kilos) + (5 X height in cm) - (6.8 X age in years)

Step 2

To determine your total daily calorie needs, now multiply your BMR by the appropriate activity factor, as follows:

Sedentary (little or no exercise): BMR X 1.2

Lightly Active (exercise/sports 1-3 days/week): BMR X 1.375

Moderately Active (exercise/sports 3-5 days/week): BMR X 1.55
Very Active (exercise/sports 6-7 days/week): BMR X 1.725

We suggest that you determine your BMR. It will give you an estimate of how much you can eat per day, but remember that the calculation will change with your age and activity level.

IT'S LIKE BALANCING YOUR CHECKBOOK

Regularly balancing your checkbook helps you stay in good financial shape. Similarly, monitoring your daily caloric intake helps you stay at your ideal weight, which keeps you in good health.

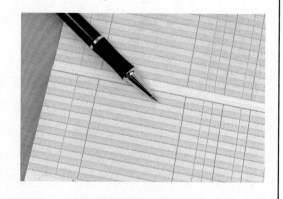

IF YOU'VE TAKEN IT OFF, YOU CAN KEEP IT OFF

If you've reached your ideal weight, you can stay there for the rest of your life by sticking with your Rice Diet program and following the guidelines we've given you in this chapter. It's normal to vary within 5 pounds of your ideal weight, but it is up to you arrest any weight gain through active intervention. It's only human to go "off the track" occasionally, but with your Rice Diet program and the maintenance information you have, you have everything you need to get back on track and stay there. As with everything else about the Rice Diet—you can do it!

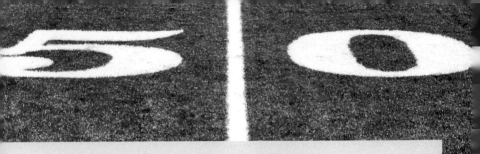

CHAPTER THIRTEEN
50 NIFTY TIPS FOR YOU

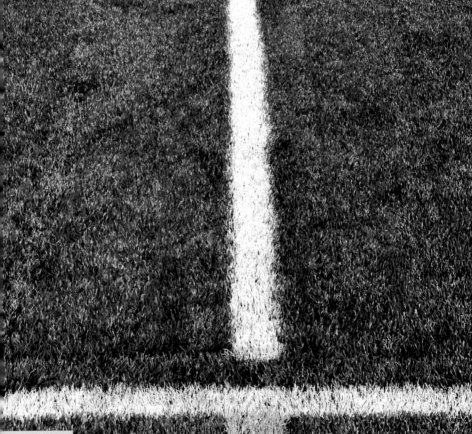

> *"To accept good advice is but to increase one's own ability."*
> —Johann Wolfgang von Goethe

WE HAVE SEEDED THE FIRST PART OF THIS BOOK WITH tips, suggestions and advice on how to succeed on your Rice Diet. The wisdom we share comes from the experience of countless Rice Dieters, and many others who have successfully met and overcome life's great challenges. To conclude Part One, we offer a list of our top 50 tips—the Nifty 50—that you can quickly and easily refer to for guidance, inspiration and direction in your quest for good health. You've learned some of these tips in previous chapters, and some you haven't, but each one of them is, in our experience, indispensable to your success. So please read them. And reread them. And re-reread them! Refer to them often and embrace them on your journey to a healthier, happier you. We offer them to you with our best wishes for your good health!

THE NIFTY 50

1. Food is not the focus of your life. Don't live to eat—eat to live!
2. Your Rice Diet is not about deprivation, it's about liberation.
3. 99% of all obesity is caused by eating too much and exercising too little. It's that simple.
4. Dieting with others makes dieting easier. Also, surround yourself with positive, supportive people.
5. The Rice Diet is a medically-based diet designed to prevent obesity, reverse and prevent disease, and maintain health.

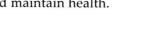

6. Consult your doctor before starting on your diet. Get a complete physical exam and blood work, including: CBC, CMP, TSH, Urine Sodium (random), Lipid Panel.
7. If you stray from your diet, get right back on it at your very next meal.
8. Check your calorie consumption and exercise routine if you hit a weight loss plateau.

9. Make daily entries in your Rice Diet Journal.

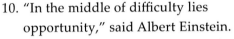

10. "In the middle of difficulty lies opportunity," said Albert Einstein.
11. Take your diet one day, one meal at a time. This makes everything much simpler and doable.
12. If you cheat on your diet, you're only cheating yourself.
13. Learn to say "No" to things that are not in your best health.
14. You can be fully satisfied with smaller portions.
15. Rice congee is versatile and filling, and has far less calories than a bowl of regular rice.

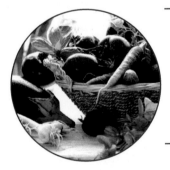

16. Rid your kitchen of unhealthy trigger foods and replace them with healthy foods and snacks.

17. Start your grocery shopping on the perimeter of the store—that's where most of the fresh produce is located.
18. Rice Diet meals and snacks are tasty, filling and healthy.

19. Cook in advance, cook more than you need, then freeze or refrigerate in small amounts for ready-to-eat meals. Remember to label and date whenever you store.
20. Salt, fat and sugar are the enemies of the Rice Diet!
21. Most commercially prepared and restaurant foods are high in sodium, fat and sugar.
22. Never eat out of a bag. Instead, remove a portion, put it on your plate and put the bag away.
23. Daily activities such as housecleaning, gardening and washing your car are beneficial physical activities too.
24. Daily weighing is a good way to avoid weight gain and regain.
25. Stress leads to feeding your emotions. Use the tips in this book to manage stress.

---

26. There are many ways to deal with phantom hunger, including:

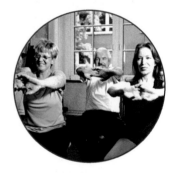

- Exercising
- Enjoying cup of tea
- Calling a friend
- Writing in your journal
- Practicing deep breathing
- Reading a book

---

27. Don't complain about having to diet. Instead celebrate the opportunity to regain your health!
28. When eating out, make the restaurant aware of your dietary needs, and insist (politely) that your food be prepared accordingly.
29. Don't let others "food push" you off your diet. No one has the right to interfere with your good health!

30. Cultivate a positive attitude about your diet and yourself. You are taking responsibility for your life, you are working to achieve your goal of health and happiness, and you can succeed with the Rice Diet.

31. Be mindful of your eating: every bite, nibble and sample contains calories.

32. Read the labels on food products to note serving size and amounts of salt, fat and sugar.

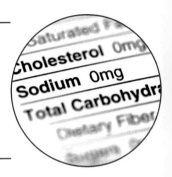

33. Products to avoid include:
- Salt
- MSG (monosodium glutamate)
- Soy sauce
- Most canned soups
- Bleu cheese and Feta cheese
- Buttered foods
- Foods in crèmes
- Gravy
- Hollandaise sauce
- Au gratin (cheese laden)
- Fried anything
- Pickles, relish, sauerkraut, mustard, ketchup (salt-free options are available)
- Salad dressings
- Skin on chicken
- Canned tomato juice
- Fatty meats
- Duck (unless fat is removed)

34. Salty foods leave you feeling hungry for more. Beware!

35. Eat slowly and stretch your meal times.

36. Drink 6 to 8 glasses of water daily, including a glass before each meal.

37. Avoid carbohydrates loaded with sugar; look for carbs that provide 2 to 3 grams of fiber per serving.

38. Snack on fruits and vegetables, not cookies and candy.

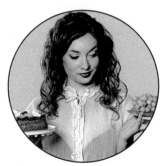

39. Saturated fat and trans fat raise cholesterol. Avoid food that boasts no cholesterol but are high in these fats.

40. Watch your calories, exercise, lose that weight.

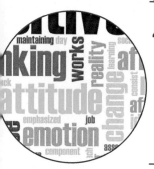

41. "I can be healthy. I can follow the Rice Diet regimen. I can lose weight and regain my health." Memorize this affirmation and say it often.

42. Serve healthy, Rice Diet-friendly foods at your holiday gatherings, and look for the same at the gatherings you attend.

43. Health problems caused by obesity have a significant impact on our nation's healthcare costs. Reversing obesity is an important national healthcare goal.

44. Lose the excuses, lose the rationalizations, and you can lose weight.

45. When done correctly, deep breathing is a quick and simple way to relax and reduce stress.

46. Reward yourself when you lose weight with new clothes for the new you.

47. For most people genuine physical hunger occurs 4 to 6 hours after the last eaten meal.

48. Trick your tummy: use small dishes and glasses for your meals.

49. You don't have to be perfect to succeed—just PERSISTENT.

50. Losing weight will make you feel better physically, emotionally and psychologically. You'll feel better— and better about yourself!

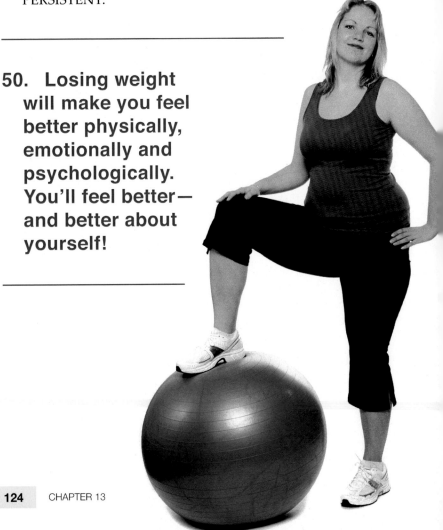

Your quest to lose weight and get healthy is both noble and necessary. The Rice Diet is your ticket to good health, but you can only succeed if you are determined, focused, sincere and serious about achieving your goals.

There can be many obstacles along your path, such as lack of knowledge about nutrition, emotional issues, food saboteurs, and more, but with motivation and determination, you can succeed.

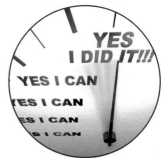

Remember to always follow the Rice Diet 10 Commandments, and be aware of the four stages of your journey:

BEFORE
When you realized that your weight problem is literally weighing you down, physically, mentally and emotionally.

DURING
The time when you are fully engaged in your Rice Diet lifestyle and working toward achieving your ideal weight.

AFTER
The period when you have achieved your ideal weight—you've won the fight, but not the war!

THEREAFTER
Once you have achieved your ideal weight, you must focus on maintaining it forever!

You are a courageous person, determined to reach for the best in yourself and the best in life. We admire you for your courage and commitment. We know you can do it!

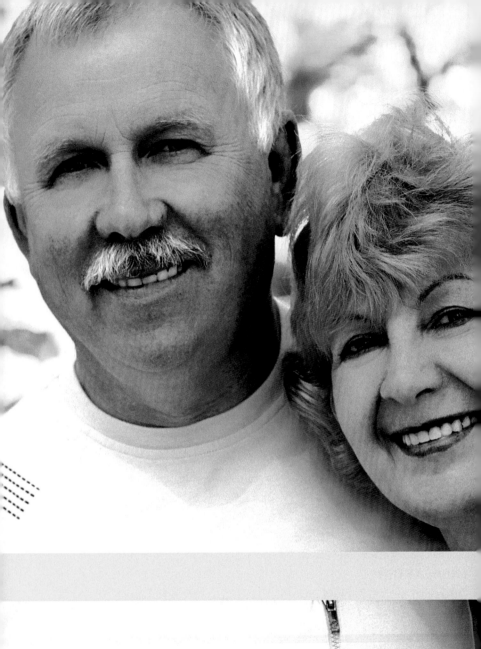

PART TWO

PART TWO
THE TOOLS FOR SUCCESS

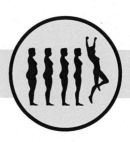

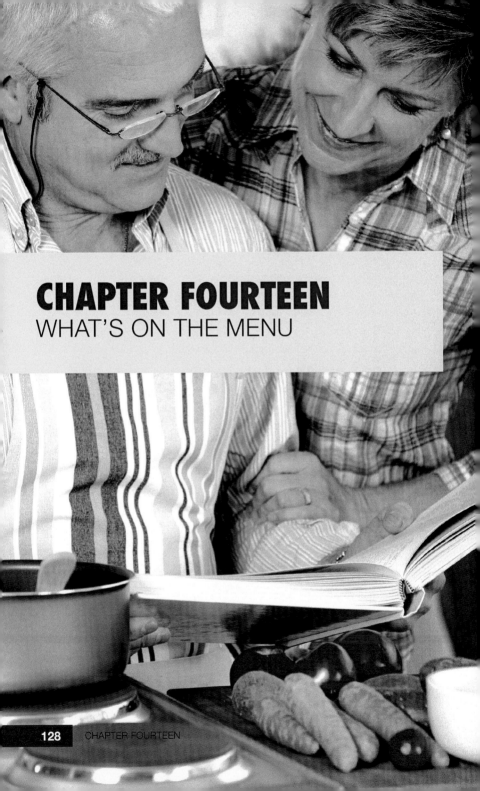

CHAPTER FOURTEEN
WHAT'S ON THE MENU

IMPORTANT

The following steps are required <u>BEFORE</u> using the Rice Diet menu:

- Consult your physician and get a complete physical exam, including the following blood work: CBC, CMP, TSH, Urine Sodium, Lipid Panel.

- DO NOT begin Week 1 of this diet if you are taking diuretics or combination anti-hypertensive–diuretic pills for high blood pressure. Ask your doctor if you are not sure about this, since using these medicines with the Week 1 diet can cause serious complications.

- If you have kidney failure of any degree, do not start this diet without first consulting your doctor. If you are taking Coumadin, your PT and INR levels may change. Your doctor must closely monitor this every 1 to 2 weeks for the first 4 to 6 weeks of your diet.

The Rice Diet menu provides tasty, filling, satisfying meals that you will enjoy eating, even as you lose weight, reverse your medical conditions and improve your health. The menu is both healthy and hearty—truly the best of both worlds! Naturally, there will be a short period of adjustment, as your body (and mind) transitions from your present diet to the Rice Diet. You'll be amazed, though, at how quickly you adjust to eating right, dropping foods high in salt, fat and processed sugar for foods that are good, and good for you. The reason for this is simple: your body reacts better to healthy, nutritious food (which is also why going back to "bad" foods causes dieters to feel lousy).

If you want your diet to work, YOU MUST STICK WITH IT!
The Rice Diet allows you to eat a wide variety of foods, but you must stick to the daily guidelines of your diet—daily. Taking a vacation from your Rice Diet is a one-way ticket back to health problems and unhappiness. **You deserve better!** And better is what you'll get by simply following your diet, day in, day out.

WEEKS ONE AND TWO
Breakfast: You may choose 1 fruit from the list on the following page plus 1 cup of beverage AND:
- 1/2 cup shredded wheat (90 calories, 0mg sodium)
- OR 2/3 cup Quaker Oats Oatmeal (100 calories, 0mg sodium)
- OR 2/3 cup Cream of Rice (100 calories, 0mg sodium)
  You may add soymilk
- OR You may have skim milk (1/2 cup, 45 calories, 60mg sodium)

Any canned fruits eaten should be in natural juice, unsweetened juice or light syrup and make certain to drain your fruit before eating.

Tips:
- You may add NO SALT tomato sauce to your 1/2 cup rice
  1/2 cup no salt tomato sauce = 15mg sodium, 30 calories
- You may use MRS. DASH (granulated or liquid form) to season your sauce or rice, limit it to 1 Tbsp = 25 calories; 0mg sodium
- You may add powdered CINNAMON to rice to get a sweet taste as desired
- You may wish to chew sugar free gum as needed; careful NOT to use too much gum that contains sorbitol, because that will cause diarrhea

Lunch: Choose 2 fruits + 1/2 cup cooked rice + 3 oz (2/3 cup) frozen or fresh vegetables (1/2 cup rice = 170 calories; if you choose to eat 3/4 cup rice = 250 calories; + 1 beverage)

Dinner: Choose 2 fruits + 1/2 cup cooked rice + 3 oz (2/3 cup) frozen or fresh vegetables (1/2 cup rice = 170 calories; if you choose to eat 3/4 cup rice = 250 calories; + 1 beverage)

Including vegetables with your meal will add 40-60mg sodium and 40-60 calories to each meal.

Allowed Rice: Brown or white, basmati, jasmine, arborio, parboiled or converted. AVOID any rice packages that appear to be commercially packaged until you check the labels; sodium should be under 10mg per cup.

Allowed Fruits:

1 orange
1 cup blueberries
1/2 cup canned peaches
1 cup pineapple, canned
1 fresh pear
1 cup unsweetened applesauce
1 cup of fresh made juice = 1 fruit
1 cup watermelon, cubed
1/2 cup sweetened applesauce
1/2 grapefruit
1/2 small cantaloupe
3 prunes
1 cup fresh strawberries
1 pomegranate
1/2 cup fruit cocktail (light syrup)
1 small banana
1/2 cup mandarin oranges

1/4 fresh honeydew
1 cup fresh cherries
3 figs
1 cup pears, unsweetened
1 cup pumpkin, canned
1/2 cup papaya, cubed
1 med-large tomato or
8 cherry tomatoes
1 apple
1 fresh peach
1/3 cup raisins
1 cup grapes
2 kiwi

Beverage Options:
Decaf coffee, tea, water, lemonade (unsweetened)
You may add crystal light with your water or artificial sweeteners such as Splenda, Truvia, or Equal.

You may add one of the following to your coffee or tea:

- Non-dairy coffee creamer - 1 tsp, 10 calories, 0mg sodium
- Westsoy Organic Unsweetened Soymilk – 1 Tbsp, 8 calories, 2mg sodium

Total fluid intake per day equals 48-64 ounces.

WEEKS THREE, FOUR, FIVE

- Refer to Week #2 Menu
- For Week #3: You may add fish or chicken/turkey in 3 oz. servings 2 times per week
- For Week #4 and #5: You may have a 3 oz. serving of fish/chicken or turkey up to 4 times per week

If there is a plateau of weight loss or weight gain at any point, go back to Week #1 menu until weight loss resumes.

NUTRITION INFORMATION FOR FISH, CHICKEN, TURKEY, MEAT

3 oz. serving	Calories	Protein	Sodium
Salmon (fresh)	150	22	50
Tuna (fresh)	118	25	39
Tuna, white, can, chunk Starkist	105	23	45
Tuna, chunk light, can, no salt	105	24	55
Salmon, Alaskan Pink, can, low sodium	120	15	75
Sardines, no salt added, 4.25 oz can	130	22	50
Chicken	186	34	76
Turkey	184	35	82
Beef	164	27	53

NEW ITEMS BEING ADDED

Tofu: Soft (silken) has the least amount of calories. It can be used as a topping when you stir it well, as a nice edition on top of the rice noodles or miracle noodles (listed below) with tomato paste, as an "ersatz ricotta topping" if this should appeal to you.

Tofu (soft/silken) serving:	*4 oz.*	*69 calories*	*9mg sodium*	*4gm fat*
Tofu (firm) serving:	*4 oz.*	*79 calories*	*14mg sodium*	*5gm fat*

Shirataki Miracle Noodle: This is a Shirataki Pasta that can be added to a meal to give it more bulk. It is made from the root of a plant called konnyaku imo. This product is available in a 7 oz. bag. Use 3.5 oz (half the bag); prepare according to package directions; mix into a rice and veggie lunch or dinner—you may add the permitted tomato sauce (refer to your list); always note your serving size and calories when preparing your meal.

Miracle Noodle serving:	*3.5 oz*	*0 calories*	*0mg sodium*	*0gm fat*

This is not a quick fix! This product, Miracle Noodle, offers no nutritional value, but can provide more bulk to your meal and make you feel full longer. You may use this as you need it.

WEEK SIX

- You may add 1 egg white per week (17 calories, 55mg sodium); if no problems with cholesterol, you may have 1 whole egg (78 calories, 62mg sodium).
- Bible Bread with Pure Honey - 8.5 oz package; 1 cracker = 43 calories; 1mg sodium; .5gm fat
- Marco Polo Golden Rusk Toast - 4 pieces = 105 calories; 5mg sodium; < 1gm fat
- Melba Toast, Old London, Salt Free, Whole Grain, 3 pieces = 60 calories; 0mg sodium; 0gm fat

Once again, if there is a plateau of weight loss or weight gain at any point, go back to Week #1 menu until weight loss resumes.

WEEK SEVEN

Ricers! You are now able to eat anything that is on the menus from weeks 1 through 6. You should follow these basic rules:

1. Average daily caloric intake should be 1000 calories (between 800-1000 calories daily).
2. Use the caloric counts you have learned along with the use of a calorie counter. Enter your daily caloric intake into your journal, in your daily food diary.
3. If you are on a plateau or gain weight, go on the week #1 menu plan until you begin to lose weight.
4. Try to do at least 1 day per week from the Week #1 menu even if you are not on a plateau.
5. As always, remember...NO SALT!!! Watch out for salt hidden in the ingredients, i.e. salad dressings, toppings, salted potatoes, wild rice, etc. Eat foods steamed, broiled, plainly grilled or boiled.

Refer to Chapter 15 for Ricer Approved Recipes. Make certain you are absolutely clear on what one serving is and what the calories, sodium and fat contents are for that one serving. Always make certain to read the nutrition (food) labels on all products!

WEEK EIGHT

Welcome to Week Eight. At this point you should be monitoring what you eat based on your weight, blood pressure and diabetic status. You may have fish or chicken or beef (beef is least favorable for anyone with heart disease, angina, cardiac stents or coronary bypass, high blood pressure or history of stroke); up to 3-4 times a week is permissible.

If you are not losing any weight, go to the Week #1 and #2 menu for two days consecutively until weight drops. Then, go to the Week #3 menu for one day, then back to the Week #4 menu. Always increase your exercise (or START doing it) if you are not losing weight. You should be trying to lose 1-3 pounds per week. Above all, watch your sodium intake. Stay below 600mg per day if possible, and NEVER go above 1000mg per day.

THERE IS NO MAGIC PILL

Remember: there is no magic pill, there is no quick fix, and dieting takes work. You have to be willing to do the work, to make adjustments and sacrifices in your daily life, to

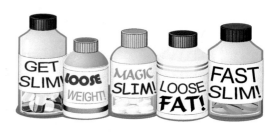

change your old ways and acquire new skills in order to achieve your goals. Give up the old habits that haven't worked and:

- Avoid the triggers that cause you to eat/cheat (routines, places)
- Rethink it—be conscious of your actions
- Magic Mantra—to stop you in your tracks, "Let it go!"
- Move it and lost it, don't sit still
- Review your journal daily and make daily entries
- Eat as prescribed based on your Rice Diet week
- Exercise routinely
- Take your daily multiple vitamin
- Seek support from others in times of compromise

Don't be a member of the yo-yo syndrome club. In order to succeed, you have to be in it for the long haul, and what that means is: slow and steady wins the race!

NUTRITION INFORMATION FOR FRUITS

Fruit	Amount	Calories	Sodium	Fiber
Apple, 1 med.	5.4 oz	80	0mg	5.0gms
Apple Juice	8.0 fl oz	80	0mg	0.0gms
Applesauce, Motts	1/2 cup	50	0mg	1.0gms
Blueberries, Fresh	1/2 cup	41	5mg	2.0gms
Blueberries, Frozen	1 cup	70	10mg	4.0gms
Cantaloupe	1/2 cup	29	7mg	0.7gms
Cranberry Juice	2 oz.	23	1mg	2.0gms
Cranberry, Fresh	1/2 cup	23	1mg	2.0gms
Grapes, Fresh	10 med. *(1.4oz)*	15	tr.	0.3gms
Honeydew melon	1 cup	60	17mg	1.0gms
Kiwi, Fresh	1 med. *(3.1oz)*	46	4mg	2.6gms
Mango, Fresh	1/2 med. *(5.3oz)*	70	0mg	1.0gms
Orange, Fresh	1 med. *(6.3oz)*	62	0mg	7.0gms
Orange Juice, Fresh	1/2 cup	56	1mg	0.3gms
Papaya, Fresh	1/2 med. *(4.9oz)*	60	10mg	2.0gms
Pomegranate	1 fresh	100	5mg	0.0gms
Raspberry, Fresh	1 cup	50	0mg	8.0gms
Strawberry, Fresh	8 med. *(5.2oz)*	45	0mg	4.0gms
Tomatoes:				
Fresh, chopped	1 cup	38	16mg	2.0gms
Canned/diced/no salt	1/2 cup	25	50mg	2.0gms
Crushed	1/4 cup	20	0mg	1.0gms
Sauce, no salt	1/4 cup	20	20mg	<1.0gms

NUTRITION INFORMATION FOR VEGETABLES

Vegetables	Amount	Calories	Sodium	Fiber
Asparagus, Fresh	5 med. *(3.3oz)*	25	0mg	2.0gms
Avocado, Fresh	1/3 med *(1.1oz)*	55	0mg	3.0gms
Avocado, Cubed	1 cup	240	11mg	10.1gms
Avocado, Pureed	1/2 cup	185	8mg	7.7gms
Broccoli	3 oz	35	45mg	2.0gms
Brussel sprouts	4 oz	30	20mg	3.5gms
Carrot	3 oz	30	60mg	2.0gms
Cauliflower	3.5 oz	25	30mg	2.0gms
Corn	4 oz	90	15mg	2.5gms
Cucumber, 8-1/4" long	1 med.	38	6mg	2.4gms
Eggplant, Fresh/cubed	1 cup	25	3mg	2.0gms
Eggplant, Fresh	1 med/1 large	60/110	5mg/10mg	
Green Beans	3 oz	20	5mg	2.0gms
Lettuce	6 oz	20	70mg	2.0gms
Mushrooms	3 oz	20	15mg	1.0gms
Onions, Fresh/chopped	1/2 cup	30	2mg	1.4gms
Peppers, Fresh/chopped:				
Red or Green	1/2 cup	20	1mg	1.3gms
Radishes	4 oz	15	15mg	1.0gms
Potato, baked/skinless	1 *(1-1/3")*	145	8mg	2.3gms
Pumpkin	4 oz	40	5mg	5.0gms
Sweet potato	3 oz	50	45mg	4.0gms
Squash, Raw, whole	1 med	39	4mg	4.0gms
Zucchini, Raw, whole	1 med	27	6mg	2.0gms

SELECTION OF PERMITTED FOODS FOR RICERS

- Cream of Rice (14 oz)

  Serving: 1 cup = 170 calories; 0 sodium; 0 fat

- Thai Kitchen Rice Noodles (14 oz)

  Serving: 2 oz = 180 calories; 0 sodium; .5gm fat

- Brown Rice Snaps – Crackers

  Serving: 8 crackers = 60 calories; 0 sodium; 0 fat

- Annie's Naturals Raspberry Vinaigrette (8 oz bottle)

  Serving: 2 Tbsp = 40 calories, 60mg sodium, 3gm fat

- 4C Totally Light Tea 2 Go (24 packets) 0 sodium, 0 calories

- Herb Ox Sodium Free Chicken or Beef Bouillon (8 packets)

  Serving: 1 packet = 10 calories; 0 sodium; 0 fat

- No Salt Added Tomato Sauce (8 oz can)

  Serving: 1/4 cup = 20 calories; 15mg sodium; 0 fat

- No Salt Added Green Beans (14.5 oz can)

  Serving: 1/2 cup = 20 calories; 15mg sodium; 0 fat

- Heinz No Salt Added Tomato Ketchup (15oz bottle)

  Serving: 1 Tbsp = 25 calories; 5mg sodium; 0 fat

- Maxwell House Lite (1/2 the caffeine) Coffee

- Westsoy Organic Unsweetened Soymilk (1 quart)

  Serving: 1 cup = 90 calories; 30mg sodium; 4.5gm fat

- Quaker Grits (Old Fashioned) (24 oz)

  Serving: 1/4 cup = 150 calories; 0 sodium; 0.5gm fat

- Old Fashioned Oats - *Serving - 1/2 cup = 150 calories; 0 sodium; 2.5gm fat*

- Quick Cooking Oats - *Serving - 1/2 cup = 140 calories; 0 sodium; 2.5gm fat*

- Edy's Fruit Bars - *Serving: 1 bar = 80 calories; 0 sodium*

- Jelly Belly Freezer Pops (Freeze & Eat) *2 oz bar = 35 calories; 0 sodium; 0 fat*

- Smucker's Low Sugar No Artificial Sweeteners Jelly, Strawberry

  Serving: 1 Tbsp = 25 calories; 0 sodium; 0 fat
- Pumpkin, canned, organic - *1/2 cup = 50 calories; 6mg sodium; 0 fat*
- Dole Tropical Fruit Salad in Lightly Sweetened Passion Fruit Juice

  Serving: 1/2 cup = 90 calories; 0 sodium; 0 fat
- Rice Cakes, unsalted, 4.5 oz package, *1 cake = 30 calories; 0 sodium, 0 fat*
- Bearitous Organic Microwave Popcorn, No Salt, No Oil; 8.4 oz package,

  Serving: 1 cup = 25 calories; 0 sodium; 1.5gm fat
- Post Shredded Wheat Original (16.4 oz box)

  Serving: 1 cup = 170 calories; 0 sodium; 1gm fat
- Dannon Light & Fit Yogurt 6 oz. container

  Serving: 2 oz. = 80 calories; .75mg sodium; 0 fat
- Kavli Crispy Thin Crackers - 5.2 oz box

  3 pieces = 50 calories; 45mg sodium, 0 fat
- Miracle Noodle, Shirataki Pasta 7oz bag; *0 calories; 0 sodium; 0 fat*
- Corn Off The Cob, unsalted (4 oz package)

  Serving: 1 oz = 105 calories; 0 sodium; 1gm fat
- Mrs. Dash Salt Free Spicy Teriyaki Marinade (12 oz bottle)

  Serving: 1 Tbsp = 25 calories; 0 sodium, .5gm fat
- Crown Prince Natural Chunk Light Tongol Tuna in Spring Water

  Serving: 1/4 cup = 70 calories; 35mg sodium; 0 fat
- Crown Prince Natural Alaskan Pink Salmon

  Serving: 1/4 cup = 80 calories; 50mg sodium; 1gm fat
- McCormick Salt Free "It's A Dilly" Seasoning; *1/4 tsp, 0 calories; 0 sodium*
- McCormick Salt Free "Spicy" Seasoning; *1/4 tsp; 0 calories; 0 sodium*
- Delmonte No Salt Added Petite Cut Diced Tomatoes

  Serving: 1/2 cup = 25 calories; 50mg sodium; 0 fat

SELECTION OF PERMITTED FOODS FOR RICERS (CONT.)

- Muir Glen Organic No Salt Added Diced Tomatoes; *1/2 cup = 30 calories; 15mg sodium; 0 fat, See label on can for excellent Salsa recipe*

- Worcestershire Sauce, World Harbors, Angostura

  Serving: 1 tsp = 5 calories; 20mg sodium; 0 fat

- White Rice Pasta, Spaghetti Style, Gluten Free; 16 oz package

  Serving: 2 oz dry = 200 calories; 0 sodium; 0 fat

- Agave Nectar (Honey); *1 Tbspp = 60 calories; 0 sodium; 0 fat*

- Oatmeal, 100% Organic Original Instant

  Serving: 1 packet = 100 calories; 0 sodium; 2gm fat

- Puffed Rice Cereal, Quaker

  Serving: 1 cup = 50 calories; 0 sodium; .1gm fat

- Pancake Syrup, Maple, Seelect Low Carb; *0 calories; 0 sodium*

- Bible Bread with Pure Honey - 8.5 oz package

  1 cracker = 43 calories; 1mg sodium; .5gm fat

- Marco Polo Golden Rusk Toast

  Serving: 4 pieces = 105 calories; 5mg sodium; < 1gm fat

- Melba Toast, Old London, Salt Free, Whole Grain

  Serving: 3 pieces = 60 calories; 0 sodium; 0 fat

- Kashi Cinnamon Harvest Cereal; *1 cup = 190 calories; 0 sodium; 1gm fat*

- Erewhon Crispy Brown Rice Cereal, Low Sodium

  Serving: 1 cup = 110 calories; 5mg sodium; 1gm fat

- Gilda Crackers No Salt or Sugar Added, A Cholesterol Free Food; 12 oz.

  Serving: 6 crackers = 140 calories; 0 sodium; 4gm fat

- Annie Chun's Rice Express Fresh Steamed Black Pearl Rice Ready in 1 Minute; Microwaveable 6.3oz package; *Serving: 1/2 tray; servings per container = 2; calories per serving = 140; 0 sodium; 1gm fat*

- Reese Imported Original Holland Rusk, light crisp toast, 3.5 oz package
  Serving: 2 pieces = 60 calories; 45mg sodium; .5gm fat
- Barbara's Crunch Organic Granola Bars Oats & Honey or Cinnamon
  7.4 oz pkg. 10 bars, *Serving: 1 bar = 95 calories; 30mg sodium; 4gm fat*
- Sweet 'N Low Gingerbread Snack Cake Mix-No Sugar Added, 8oz package
  Makes 5 servings; Serving: 1/5 package = 160 calories; 30mg sodium; 2.5gm fat
- Streit's Unsalted Matzos, 11oz package
  Serving: 1 matzo = 100 calories; 0 sodium; 0 fat
- Westbrae Natural Stoneground Mustard No Salt Added; 8 oz container
  Serving: 1 teaspoon = 0 calories; 0 sodium; 0 fat
- Farmer Boy Restaurant House Recipe Greek Dressing 16 oz. bottle,
  Serving: 2 Tbsp = 25 calories; 10mg sodium; 2gm fat (this version only)
- Consorzio Mango Fat-Free Dressing; 12 fluid oz. bottle
  Serving: 1 Tbsp = 10 calories; 10mg sodium; 0 fat
- Maple Grove Farms of Vermont Maple Fig All Natural Dressing
  12 oz. fluid oz. bottle - *Serving: 2 Tbsp = 30 calories; 0 sodium; 0 fat*
- Rice Road All Natural Sweet & Sour Sauce with Peanuts-Low Sodium;
  8 fluid oz. bottle - *Serving: 1 Tbsp = 30 calories; 35mg sodium; 0gm fat*
- Mr. Spice Organic Salt Free Thai Peanut Sauce & Marinade;
  10.5 fluid oz. bottle - *Serving: 1 Tbsp = 25 calories; 0 sodium; 1gm fat*
- Mr. Spice Organic Honey Mustard Sauce & Marinade; 10.5 fluid oz. bottle
  Serving: 1 Tbsp = 35 calories; 0 sodium; 0 fat
- Mr. Spice Organic Salt Free Indian Curry Sauce & Marinade;
  10.5 fluid oz. bottle - *Serving: 1 Tbsp = 15 calories; 0 sodium; 0 fat*
- Mr. Spice Organic Salt Free Honey BBQ and Marinade; 10.5 fluid oz.
  bottle - *Serving: 2 Tbsp = 40 calories; 0 sodium; 0 fat*
- Mr. Spice Organic Salt Free Sweet & Sour Sauce & Marinade
  10.5 fluid oz. bottle - *Serving: 2 Tbsp = 45 calories; 0 sodium; 0 fat*

- Alberto's Sweet Jalapeño Relish Sweet and Tangy-Mild; 13.5 oz jar

  Serving: 2 Tbsp = 30 calories; 0 sodium; 0 fat

- Tomatillo Garlic Salsa Just A Tad Hot; 12 oz. jar

  Serving: 2 Tbsp = 20 calories; 15mg sodium; 0 fat

- Sweet 'N Low Pancake Mix, Sugar Free, Fat Free, Cholesterol-Free Low

  Sodium, Just add water; 8 oz. box; makes 5 servings

  Serving: 1/5 package = 150 calories; 20mg sodium; 0 fat

- Santa Barbara SALSA Mango with Peach

  Serving: 1 Tbsp = 10 calories; 43mg sodium; 0 fat

- Delmonte No Sugar Added Mandarin Oranges in sweetened water,

  15 oz can - *Serving: 1/2 cup = 45 calories; 10mg sodium; 0 fat*

- Apple Butter Fruit Spread, Walden Farms, Calorie Free, 12 oz jar;

  Serving: 1 Tbsp = 0 calories; 0 sodium; 0 fat

- Blueberry Fruit Spread, Walden Farms, Calorie Free, 12 oz jar;

  Serving: 1 Tbsp = 0 calories; 0 sodium; 0 fat

- Cool Whip LITE: 12 oz. tub; *2 Tbsp = 20 calories; 0 sodium; 1gm fat*

- Marshmallow Dip, Walden Farms, Calorie Free, 12 oz jar;

  Serving: 1 Tbsp = 0 calories; 25mg sodium; 0 fat

- Caramel Dip, Walden Farms, Calorie Free, 12 oz jar

  Serving: 1 Tbsp = 0 calories; 10mg sodium; 0 fat

- Peanut Spread, Whipped, Walden Farms, Calorie Free, Creamy; 12 oz jar

  Serving: 1 Tbsp = 0 calories; 53mg sodium; 0 fat

- Alfredo Sauce, Walden Farms, Calorie Free, 15 oz jar;

  Serving: 3 Tbsp = 0 calories; 20mg sodium; 0 fat

- LaChoy Fancy Bamboo Shoots, in water, 8 oz can

  Serving: 1/2 cup = 10 calories; 10mg sodium; 0 fat

- Smart Balance buttery spread light with flax oil

  Serving: 2 tsp 32 calories; 54mg sodium; 3gm fat
- Veg-all original mixed vegetables, no salt added, 15 oz can;

  Serving: 1/2 cup = 40 calories; 25mg sodium; 0 fat
- Health Valley Organic, no salt added, Tomato Soup 15 oz can;

  Serving: 1 cup = 100 calories; 60mg sodium; 2.5gm fat
- Health Valley Organic, no salt added, Mushroom Barley soup 15 oz can;

  Serving: 1 cup = 90 calories; 60mg sodium; 2.5gm fat

HEALTHY SUBSTITUTIONS

- Dannon Light & Fit yogurt, FAGE or OIKOS Greek Yogurt All Natural 0% Fat instead of sour cream
- Sorrento Part Skim Ricotta Cheese (in moderation)
- Applesauce instead of butter or oil
- Friendship salt-free cottage cheese in place of other cottage cheese
- Crumbles instead of ground beef
- Some Fluff with a banana instead of Boston Cream Pie
- Lite Cherry Pie Filling with Cool Whip instead of Cherry Pie and whipped cream
- Pumpkin (with pumpkin pie spice) and Cool Whip instead of Pumpkin Pie
- Edy's Fruit Bars or Jelly Belly Freezer Pops instead of ice cream
- Dannon Lite & Fit Yogurt, FAGE or Stonyfield Oilos Plain Greek Yogurt instead of sour cream or ice cream
- Pancake Syrup, Maple, Seelect Low Carb, dip for apple slices, bananas, orange, pear
- Caramel Dip, Walden Farms, Calorie Free
- Feather Weight Baking Powder Sodium Free, Gluten Free

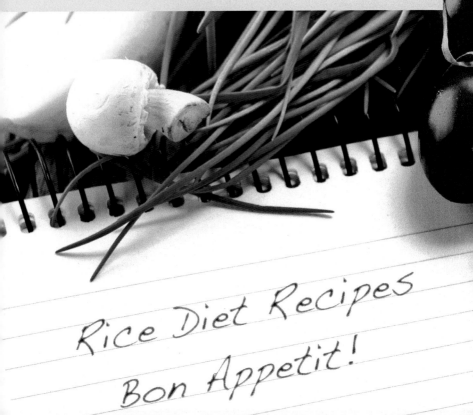

CHAPTER FIFTEEN
RECIPES

Rice Diet Recipes

Bon Appetit!

FEAST YOUR EYES ON ALL THE DELICIOUS MEALS and snacks you can enjoy on the Rice Diet. There's no end to all the good things you can eat, and once you get started, you'll see why so many Ricers say, "I've never eaten better in my life!"

CREATIVE COOKING IDEAS

1. In a blender, puree an assortment of vegetables (peppers, carrots, onions, tomatoes, mixed vegetables, squash, etc.). Add Mrs. Dash or teaspoon of no sodium mustard, or add no sodium tomato sauce. Heat this mixture and pour over cooked rice or rice noodles, a plain baked potato, fish or chicken.

2. Canned pumpkin makes a wonderful dessert: sprinkle contents of can with cinnamon, 2 packets of Splenda, add some Seelect pancake maple syrup if desired. Calories: 140; 1/2 cup = 40 calories

3. Add fruit to your salad, throw in some raisins, cut up apples or slices of orange for a change in taste and texture.

4. Add shredded cabbage (found in grocery stores in bags labeled "for cole slaw"), to no sodium salad dressings, or when cooking soup, or heat in a small amount of water (on stove or in a covered, microwave-safe bowl) until the desired crispness. Start out with 2 minutes at high temperature, stir, cook more if desired.

5. Refer to the RICER SALSA recipe you were given and serve on baked potatoes or fish.

6. Puree silken tofu as a substitute for mayonnaise in recipes, or blend with frozen fruit (ex. blueberries). Add Splenda if desired for your own homemade yogurt!

7. Fresh mushrooms: eat them plain, in salads, with rice, or with no sodium dressing—healthy and low in calories.

HELPFUL TIPS FOR EASY ACCESS SNACKS

Why not purchase a tray with a lid, in plastic, available in most stores. It has compartments and you can place items in it for "easy grasp." Have foods readily available whenever you feel the need to eat something; you might as well eat something healthy and guilt free! Depending on foods, place in the refrigerator or on the counter top.

Here's some suggested foods you can use:

- Frozen Blueberries
- Cucumbers
- Kashi Lean and Crunchy Cereal
- Lite cherry pie filling
- Apple Slices
- Baby Carrots
- Applesauce
- Frozen Grapes

- Banana
- Cool Whip-Lite
- Pumpkin from can
- Almonds-unsalted
- Dannon Lite and Fit yogurt
- Marshmallow Fluff
- Various Fruits
- Various Vegetables

The following 34 pages are filled with original recipes compiled by Denise Sprung. They are designed to be easy and quick to produce, even for the novice cook. These are recipes that have been created for the "Ricers" attending the Rice Diet of Central Florida program.

BEVERAGES

✳ **DIET CRANBERRY BEVERAGE AVAILABLE IN STORES**
No artificial flavorings or preservatives.
Ingredients: Filtered water, concentrated cranberry juice, natural flavors, pectin, citric acid, fumaric acid, sucralose (23mg / 250mL), sodium citrate, acesulfame potassium (40mg / 250mL), ascorbic acid (vitamin C), color. *Calories per 1/2 cup serving: 35.* Create your own low-calorie beverage with the suggestions below:

Spritzerberry: 6 ounces Ocean Spray® Light Cranberry Juice Drink or Diet Ocean Spray® Juice Drink, any flavor, 2 ounces diet ginger ale or sparkling water. Pour all ingredients in a tall glass over ice. Makes 1 serving.

Mixed Berry Smoothie: 3/4 cup Ocean Spray® Light Cranberry Juice Drink or Diet Ocean Spray® Juice Drink, any flavor, 3/4 cup frozen mixed berries (strawberries, raspberries, blackberries and blueberries), one 6-ounce container low fat berry-flavored yogurt, 1/2 banana. Cut into slices.

Combine all ingredients in a blender. Blend for a few seconds on high speed or until ingredients are thoroughly combined. Pour into a large glass. Makes approximately 2 servings.

Low Calorie Cosmo: 3 ounces Ocean Spray® Light Cranberry Juice Cocktail or Diet Ocean Spray® Cranberry, 3/4 ounce Absolut® Raspberri® Raspberry Flavored Vodka, squeeze of lime, lime twist as a garnish. Shake ingredients (except the lime twist) until cold, in a cocktail shaker with ice. Strain into a chilled glass. Garnish with lime twist. Makes 1 serving that's just 50 calories.

GRAINS

THE BASIC QUINOA RECIPE

This light and wholesome grain may be prepared quickly and easily with this basic method: 2 cups water, 1 cup quinoa. Place quinoa and water in a 1 1/2 quart saucepan and bring to a boil. Reduce to a simmer, cover and cook until all the water is absorbed (about 15 minutes).

You will know that the quinoa is done when all the grains have turned from white to transparent, and the spiral-like germ has separated. *Makes 3 cups.*

To prepare in a rice cooker: Simply treat quinoa like rice. Add 2 parts water to 1 part quinoa, stir, cover (unlike rice, you can stir quinoa a few times while cooking to prevent burning in the bottom of the pan) and when the cooker shuts off, the quinoa is done.

Microwave Instructions: 1 cup quinoa, 2 cups water in a 2 quart microwave bowl. Cook on high 100% for 5 minutes and 60% for 8 minutes. Let stand for a few minutes and voila, perfect quinoa.

For an energy saving method, combine 1-cup water to each 1/2 cup of quinoa in a pan. Bring to a full boil for 5 minutes, and set aside covered, for 15 minutes.

For additional flavor, add Herb Ox sodium free chicken bouillon to the water in any of the methods listed above.

Ancient Harvest Quinoa has already been washed with pure water and solar dried to remove the natural bitter saponin coating.

✳ QUINOA HOT BREAKFAST CEREAL

Bring 2 cups water to a boil, add 1 cup quinoa, reduce heat, simmer 5 minutes. Add 1/2 cup thinly sliced apples, 1/4 cup raisins, 1/2 tsp cinnamon and simmer until water is absorbed. You may sweeten with Seelect No-Sodium, No-Sugar Maple Syrup, Splenda, Cinnamon, Polaner or Smuckers Sugar-Free Low-Sodium Preserves.

Our demonstration:
1 box Quinoa
4 oz can no salt added mushrooms, drained
15 oz can Eden Organic No Sodium Kidney Beans
1 container of Tomato Trinity Mix
8 oz chopped tomatoes, peppers and onions
4 cups water

Place all the above in a rice cooker. When cooking is completed you may add 1 Tbsp olive oil and 2 packets of dry herb ox Sodium Free Chicken or Beef Bouillon.

Per Serving (1/4 cup dry): Calories 172, Calories from Fat 25, Total Fat 2.8g, Saturated Fat 0g, Trans Fat 0g, Cholesterol 0mg, Sodium 1mg, Carbohydrate 31g, Dietary Fiber 3g, Soluble 36%, In-Soluble 64%, Sugars 3g, Protein 6g

✳ 10 SENSIBLE RICER SNACKS

1. When you're in a crunch, on the run, take a crunch out of a piece of fruit to fill you up, give you the energy you need and hold you over until you have your meal.
2. Make a Simple Fruit Slushie: 1 cup fresh fruit, 1/2 cup low calorie (diet)

fruit juice, 1 cup ice. Place into a blender and liquefy. Two servings.

3. Fresh fruit in bowls are a great way to satisfy cravings. Keep them readily available at home in the kitchen, work and always take along for a snack when on the run, in your car, while walking.

4. Freeze grapes, blueberries and banana slices for slow going snacking.

5. Cut up cantaloupe into small chunks and leave in refrigerator for munching on.

6. Single serving cups of All Natural Mott's applesauce. Add some blueberries.

7. 3 whole wheat no-sodium Melba Toast in Ziploc bag

8. 2 no-sodium, no-sugar Gilda crackers in Ziploc bag

9. 12 raw shelled almonds in Ziploc bag, (don't eat all at once, but throughout the day)

10. 2 cups chopped cucumber, eaten with a small fork, no-sodium dressing added

SOUPS

TOMATO-VEGETABLE SOUP

Use the Rice Diet Tomato Sauce as a base. Add any vegetables cut into small cubes or small pieces. Cook over a low heat until the vegetables are tender. If the soup is too thick, merely add water while cooking until it reaches the desired consistency. 1 cup = 1 serving.

VEGETABLES BECOME SOUP

You can make soup directly from the vegetables simply by cooking them until they are soft, then pureeing them in a food processor. Potatoes, broccoli, cauliflower, to name a few, work well. Thin the puree with water if you wish. 1 cup = 1 serving.

RICER MUSHROOM BARLEY VEGETABLE SOUP

1 15-oz can Health Valley Organic No Salt Added Mushroom Barley Soup
2 packets of Herb-ox Sodium Free Beef Bouillon
2 cups water

15-oz can Veg-All Original Mixed Vegetables No Salt Added

2 cups cooked Brown Rice (or other cooked rice)

15-oz can Eden Organic Kidney Beans No Sodium Added Fat Free

1/2 package (4-oz) of 8-oz Incredible Fresh Tri Pepper Mix

1/2 package (4-oz) of 8-oz Incredible Fresh Trinity Mix

2 cups (of a 10-oz package) Fresh Express Fine Shred Cabbage

8-oz package white sliced mushrooms

You may add any of the following ingredients according to taste preference: garlic, onions, 2 fresh chopped tomatoes, Mrs. Dash, Turmeric, Cumin, Curry, Dill. Place all ingredients in a large pot. Stir. Heat for approximately 15 minutes. Add other spices according to taste. If you wish, you may add 3 oz. of cooked crumbled chicken (without skin) if you are in the Rice Diet phase permitted you to incorporate lean fish, chicken or meat in your regimen. However, remember to add on the calories of any other product you add to the soup. *Makes 10 servings.*

Per Serving (1 cup): Calories 150, Sodium 30mg

✱ RICER BARLEY AND BEAN VEGETABLE SOUP WITH CRUMBLES

11 oz. box Quaker quick pearled barley

2 packages marjon tofu crumbles

2 cans Del Monte No Salt Added diced tomatoes

1 Tbsp Mrs. Dash

5 cups organic frozen mixed vegetables

1 tsp garlic powder

1 cup chopped onion

6 packages Herb Ox sodium free beef bouillon

1 Tbsp basil

15 oz. can no salt added pinto beans, drained

Place 12 cups of water in a very large pot on the stove. Heat the water until almost boiling and mix all the ingredients except beans and frozen vegetables, to be added later. Cover pot, bring to a boil. Reduce heat; simmer 10 minutes; stir periodically. Add drained beans and frozen vegetables, cover, continue cooking at the simmer setting for approximately 15 minutes or until the vegetables are tender. Add more water if the soup is too thick. *Makes 21 cups.*

Per Serving (1 cup): Calories 113, Fat 1.3gm, Sodium 36.7mg

FRUITS

RICER FRUIT FONDUE
2 Tbsp Dannon Light & Fit Yogurt (25 calories, 25 mg sodium)
2 Tbsp applesauce (sweetened or unsweetened) (25 calories, 0 mg sodium)
Applesauce (sweetened) 1/2 cup = 110 calories, 0 mg sodium
Mix together to use as a dip for fruits (add cinnamon if desired):
sliced apple (peeled), sliced banana, strawberries, pineapple chunks, grapes, papaya

RICER BREAKFAST PARFAIT
Place in a drinking glass (to layer items):
1/2 cup rice congee or Cream of Rice, Cream of Wheat or Quaker Oats (congee can be made in your rice cooker or by adding 1/4 cup hot water to 1/2 cup cooked rice)
1 cup fruit of choice in chunks
Put 2 Tbsp Dannon Light & Fit Yogurt on top
Add a few raisins and/or cinnamon if desired

MAPLE FRUIT OATMEAL RICE DISH
2 ripe bananas mashed with fork
2 cups drained/rinsed canned tropical fruit
2 cups cooked rice
1-1/2 cups uncooked oatmeal
2 Tbsp select maple syrup

1 chopped raw apple
2 Tbsp raisins
2 cups of water
Cinnamon, Splenda, Vanilla (1/4 tsp each and 1 packet splenda)

Thoroughly mix all the ingredients, cover, place in microwave oven for approximately 4 minutes, then stir, recover and continue cooking for another 4 minutes or until desired consistency. *Makes 8 servings.*

Per Serving: Calories 164, Fat .5gm, Sodium .9mg

✳ RICER ORANGE MAPLE CINNAMON BANANA SLICES

4 bananas peeled, sliced (approximately 50 slices)
1 Tbsp cinnamon
2 Tbsp Seelect Maple Pancake Syrup
1 Tbsp Smuckers No Sugar Orange Marmalade (or other flavor)

Place all banana slices, flat, in a freezer safe dish. Combine the other ingredients, mix well and gently brush/spoon onto the banana slices. Place in the freezer. You may add a teaspoon of Mott's Natural Applesauce on the slices for added taste. *Makes 5 servings.*

Per Serving (10 slices): Calories 76 (7.6 per slice)

✳ RICER TRIFLE-FULL OF FRUIT AND FLAVOR!

2-1/2 cups Kashi GO LEAN Crunch Cereal, divided
2 15 oz. cans Delmonte Fruit Cocktail "light"
1 apple, chopped into small pieces, divided
2 6 oz. containers Lemon Chiffon Yogurt, fat free, light
2 Tbsp Walden Farms Maple Syrup (optional)
2 cups cooked rice
2 bananas, in slices, divided
2 cups fresh blueberries, divided
10 oz. Comstock LITE Cherry Pie Filling

1 Tbsp cinnamon
1 Tbsp vanilla extract (optional)

Take a large bowl and mix the 2 cups cooked rice with the 2 cans of fruit cocktail. Add the cinnamon and vanilla extract (optional) and 2 tablespoons of maple syrup. Divide this mixture into 3 portions to be layered into a bowl. Place 1-1/2 cups of Kashi on the bottom of the bowl. Spoon 1/3 of the rice fruit mixture on top of the Kashi. The next layer is the sliced banana. Place 1/2 of the chopped apple on top of the banana slices. Add 1 cup blueberries. Gently spread 1 container of the lemon yogurt on top of the blueberries, smoothing it all around to the edges of the bowl. Now add the next 1/3 rice fruit mixture (this is the second layer). Place 1/2 can (10oz) of the cherry lite pie filling on top of the rice fruit mixture to the edges of the bowl to define the layers. The next layer will be the remaining chopped apples. Add the remaining 1 cup of blueberries on top of the apples. Add the last 1/3 rice fruit mixture on top of the blueberries. Add the remaining 1/2 can of cherry lite pie filling then place the second banana, in slices on top of the cherries. Layer the second 6oz container of the lemon yogurt on top of the banana slices. Sprinkle the remaining 1 cup of Kashi on top of the yogurt. Cover the bowl and refrigerate for several hours or overnight. But if you have to eat it right away, dig in! Enjoy your trifley good food! *Makes 12 servings.*

Per Serving (1 cup): Calories 165, Fat .7gm, Sodium 46mg

SPICY APPLE SLICES - SUPER SNACK
1 14 oz bag Crunch Pak Sweet Apple Slices
1 Tbsp Smart Balance whipped low sodium spread, melted
2 Tbsp Seelect Maple Pancake Syrup
1 Tbsp lemon juice (sprinkle over apple slices)
3 tsp Splenda Brown Sugar Blend
1/4 tsp ground nutmeg plus 1/4 tsp ground cinnamon

In a large ziplock bag or container, thoroughly mix all the above contents into snack size ziplock bags for storing your snacks. Sprinkle lemon juice onto apple slices to prevent them from browning and set aside. Soften the Smart Balance by stirring or place in microwave for a few seconds on a lower power to soften/melt, but not burn. Add ALL the above contents into a large ziplock bag (carefully make certain to zip the back shut) or use a container with a lid and gently shake contents to coat all the apple slices before placing into the microwave.

Place contents into microwave, cover with microwave lid or a paper towel for approximately 3-5 minutes, until the desired crispness. Allow to cool or refrigerate and VOILA, a spicy tasty snack to carry around in a snack size Ziploc bag. ENJOY! *Makes 24 apple slices (equivalent to 2 apples).*

Per Serving (6 slices): Calories 80, Fat 1.75gm, Sugar 18mg

VEGETABLES

✳ DIRECT GRILLING VEGETABLES: DELICIOUS AND NUTRITIOUS

Direct grilling is a great way to enjoy vegetables.

Step 1—Rinse, trim and chop your vegetables (see below for directions).

Step 2—Bring a small amount of water to a boil in a saucepan, add desired vegetables and simmer, covered (see below for specified times).

Step 3—Drain pan and brush vegetables with olive oil. Place vegetables on a piece of heavy foil or directly on the grill rack. If using a charcoal grill, place vegetables on rack directly over medium coals. Grill for directed time, or until vegetables are crisp-tender. For a gas grill—Preheat grill, then reduce heat to medium. Place vegetables on grill rack directly over heat. Cover grill. Monitor grilling closely so vegetables don't char.

Asparagus

Preparation: Bend an asparagus until it snaps naturally at the base. Discard the shorter, stem base, and use the remaining stalk as a guide to chop the rest to the appropriate length. Precook, then tie in bundles with strips of cooked green onion tops.

Precook time: 3 minutes
Direct grill time: 3-5 minutes

Baby carrots
Preparation: Cut off tops. Wash and peel.
Precook time: 3-5 minutes
Direct grill time: 3-5 minutes

Corn on the cob
Preparation: Peel back husks but do not remove. Remove silks. Rinse corn; pat dry. Fold husks back around cobs. Tie husk tops with 100%-cotton kitchen string.
Precook time: Do not precook
Direct grill time: 25-30 minutes

Eggplant
Preparation: Cut off top and blossom ends. Cut eggplant crosswise into 1-inch slices.
Precook time: Do not precook
Direct grill time: 8 minutes

Fennel
Preparation: Snip off feathery leaves. Cut off stems.
Precook time: 10 minutes; then cut into 6-8 wedges
Direct grill time: 8 minutes

Leeks
Preparation: Cut off green tops; trim bulb roots and remove 1 or 2 layers of white skin. Rinse to remove any dirt.
Precook time: 10 minutes or until almost tender; then halve lengthwise
Direct grill time: 5 minutes

New potatoes
Preparation: Scrub potatoes; pierce skin with a fork. Wrap individually in a double layer of foil.

Precook time: Do not precook
Direct grill time: 1-2 hours

Sweet peppers
Preparation: Remove stems. Halve peppers lengthwise. Remove seeds and membranes. Cut into 1-inch-wide strips.
Precook time: Do not precook
Direct grill time: 8-10 minutes

Tomatoes
Preparation: Remove cores; cut in half crosswise
Precook time: Do not precook
Direct grill time: 5 minutes

Zucchini or yellow summer squash
Preparation: Wash; cut off ends quarter lengthwise
Precook time: Do not precook
Direct grill time: 5-6 minutes

✳ RICER RATATOUILLE SPREAD
1 medium eggplant (8-1/2" x 1-3/8") chopped
(1 cup chopped = 21 calories)
Chopped version add 2-4 Tbsp of Ricer Salsa, place on top of 1/2 cup warm cooked rice OR slice eggplant (toast or grill if desired)
Distribute 2-4 Tbsp of Ricer Salsa on top of up to 6 slices of eggplant

✳ POTATO-RICE CAKES
Peel 1 medium potato and boil until soft. Add 2 Tbsp chopped onion to 2 Tbsp cooked rice and mash together. Form into patties and place on pan that has been lightly sprayed with a nonstick vegetable spray product such as Pam. Cook in a 450 degree oven until brown on the bottom, then turn over and bake until other side is brown.

BAKED ONIONS WITH TOMATOES

Cover a rectangular baking sheet with foil and spray with a nonstick vegetable spray, such as Pam. Thinly slice 2 small onions and place in a layer on top of the foil. Cover with 1/2 cup Rice Diet Tomato Sauce and sprinkle with a salt-free sweetener if desired. Bake in a 450 degree oven until it is hot and crusty; you may broil this dish if you prefer.

POTATO CHIPS

Bake or boil a medium sized potato until it can easily be pierced with a fork. Slice into a pan sprayed with a nonstick vegetable spray, such as Pam. Place under the broiler until tops are brown. Turn over and brown the other sides.
OR
Use a raw potato that has been washed and dried. Slice thin, lay the slices in a single layer on a sheet of aluminum foil sprayed with Pam. Sprinkle with Mrs. Dash if you like. Bake in a 450 degree oven for 20 minutes or until browned to your preference.

RICER POTATO CHIPS FROM POTATOES MADE IN MICROWAVE

10 medium sized red potatoes
1 Tbsp olive oil
2 Tbsp Mrs. Dash Seasoning
1 large plate to cook the potato slices on
1 large Ziploc bag to shake all items in

Wash the potatoes and dry thoroughly. Carefully secure the potato with a fork at the end and begin to slice very thin slices, approximately 1/8" thick. Each potato should yield approximately 10-12 slices. Place all the potato slices into a large Ziploc bag. Pour the 1 Tbsp of olive oil into the bag along with 2 Tbsp Mrs. Dash seasoning. Zip the bag closed and make sure it is tightly shut. Proceed to shake the ingredients, making sure to coat all the potatoes evenly with the oil and seasoning. Add slices, single layered onto a microwave-safe plate. Be sure they are in a single layer. Cook on high uncovered for approximately 3 minutes. Carefully remove the hot plate and turn the slices over. Return to the microwave for approximately

3 more minutes. Check to see if they are nicely browned and crisp. They will become a bit crisper as they cool, but you don't want them soggy in the middle, and may require another minute or two more cooking. They should feel crisp and not burnt. Remove the cooked potatoes, put onto another dish to cool and proceed with making another single layered batch on the plate to then repeat the cooking process. Store the "chips" in an airtight bag or container. *Makes 10-12 servings*

Per Serving (10-12 chips): Calories 120, Fat .01gm, Sodium 0mg
To prepare recipe for 1 person, just cook 1 potato and adjust to 1/8 tsp olive oil and a dash of Mrs. Dash.

✱ RICER CRUNCHY COLESLAW

16 oz. bag coleslaw mix (shredded green and red cabbage with carrots)
3/4 cup Fage total 0% nonfat all natural greek yogurt
1-2 packets of Splenda, according to taste
1 tsp dill weed
10 oz. can pineapple tidbits in 100% pineapple juice, drained
1/2 cup raisins
2 Tbsp Westbare no salt added stoneground mustard
3 tsp apple cider vinegar

Place coleslaw, drained pineapple and raisins in a large container. In a separate container mix yogurt, Splenda, dill weed, mustard and apple cider vinegar. Mix the dressing thoroughly, then stir into the coleslaw mixture. Either stir the entire contents until blended OR cover the container securely and while holding the top down tightly, gently shake the entire contents to thoroughly coat the coleslaw. Refrigerate for several hours before serving. *Makes 9 cups.*

Per Serving (1 cup): Calories 68, Fat 0gm, Sodium 15mg, Sugar .8g

SAUCY MUSHROOM TOFU RICE PEPPER

1 package Nasoya Lite Silken Tofu
1 package Marjon Tofu Crumbles
8 oz. package white sliced fresh mushrooms
29 oz. can tomato puree
14.5 oz. can Delmonte diced tomatoes basil, garlic, oregano, no salt added
2-1/2 cups cooked rice
Add Mrs. Dash or other desired spices according to taste
8 medium raw green peppers

Puree silken tofu in blender. Pour into microwave-safe large bowl. Add the remaining ingredients, except for the peppers, stirring very well until everything is completely mixed together. Heat on high for 5 minutes or until desired temperature. Cut tip off of each pepper. Set peppers onto microwave-safe plate with 2 tablespoons water. Spoon mixture into each pepper. If there is remainder, use on top of veggies or baked potato for other meals. Cover peppers with paper towel. Heat on high in microwave for 4 minutes. Heat longer if necessary. *Makes 8 servings.*

Per Serving (1 cup): Calories 215, Fat 2gm, Sodium 92mg

GREEN BEAN RICER CASSEROLE

14.5 oz. can No Salt Green Beans, drained
1 can LaChoy Fancy Bamboo Shoots in water, drained
1 Tbsp minced dehydrated onions
1/2 cup Walden Farms Calorie Free Alfredo Sauce
1 can no salt mushrooms Pennsylvania Dutch, drained
1/2 cup Corn Off The Cob plain, unsalted
1 Tbsp Mrs. Dash

Combine all ingredients in a large microwave safe bowl. Microwave on HIGH for approximately 3 minutes or until the desired temperature. Green bean casserole has always been a traditional recipe for the holidays, make it a nutritious one! *3 1/2 cups makes 7 servings; 1/2 cup makes 1 serving.*

Per Serving (1/2 cup): Calories 28; Fat .10gm, Sodium 18mg

✳ RICER "SWEET" WHIPPED SWEET POTATOES

4 medium sized sweet potatoes, punctured (approximately 1.5 pounds in weight total)
1/4 cup Seelect Maple Pancake Syrup
1/4 tsp cinnamon
1/2 cup Mott's Natural No Sugar Added Applesauce
15 oz. can Delmonte No Sugar Added Mandarin Oranges, reserving 1/4 cup of liquid from the can
2 Tbsp Marshmallow Fluff

Rinse the potatoes and puncture them several times. On a microwave-safe dish, cook on HIGH for approximately 13 minutes (check the potatoes after 10 minutes to see if they are thoroughly cooked). Once soft, cut in half, scrap pulp away from skin, and discard the skins. Mash with a whisk or fork, adding the other ingredients one at a time, mixing until you reach a smooth consistency. Serve hot, warm or cold. Tastes even better the next day! *4 cups makes 8 servings; 1/2 cup makes 1 serving.*

Per Serving (1/2 cup): Calories 86, Fat .05gm, Sodium 17mg

✳ SPICY STEAK FRIES

2 large potatoes
2 Tbsp no sodium spicy seasoning blend
2 Tbsp olive oil
1 clove garlic, minced

Wash and cut potatoes into wedges (do not peel). Pat dry with paper towels. In a large bowl, toss potatoes with spicy seasoning blend, olive oil and garlic. Spray baking sheet with no-stick cooking spray and lay wedges on baking sheet. Place potatoes in preheated 425 degree oven and bake for 20 minutes. Turn the potatoes and lightly spray with no-stick cooking spray. Bake another 15 minutes or until wedges are browned and tender. *Makes 4 servings.*

Per Serving (1/2 potato): Calories 200, Total Fat 7gm, Sodium 10mg

EASY PEAPODS AND PEPPERS

1/2 Tbsp Mrs. Dash Original Blend
3 cups fresh peapods
1/2 cup chopped red pepper

Cook and stir peapods and red peppers in a non-stick skillet sprayed with no-stick cooking spray over medium-high heat for 5 minutes. Stir in Mrs. Dash Original Blend and continue cooking for 2-3 minutes or until tender. *Makes 4 servings.*

Per Serving (3/4 cup): Calories 25, Total Fat 0gm, Sodium 0mg

EGGPLANT SELECTION

Today, eggplants (called aubergine in France) come in all shapes, from small, round fruits (about two inches in diameter) to the popular large oblong Black Beauty variety, which can range up to 12 inches long. A newer variety (called Japanese eggplant) is long and thin, resembling zucchini, and has fewer seeds. (The seeds are edible in all varieties.)

Eggplant colors range from white to lavender to dark purplish-black as well as pale green, yellow, and reddish. There are even some striped varieties. Various eggplant varieties may be used interchangeably in most recipes, unless the skin color is a specific visual factor in the dish.

Although available year-round, prime time for eggplant is August and September in the United States. Look for eggplants with smooth, shiny skin, heavy for their size, and no blemishes, tan patches, or bruises. Wrinkled, loose skin is an indication of age, and the fruit will be more bitter. Smaller eggplants have fewer seeds, thinner skin, and tend to be sweeter, more tender, and less bitter.

Press your finger lightly against the skin. If it leaves a light imprint, it is ripe. If it is too soft, it is too old and will be bitter. Looking for less seeds? Check the blossom end of the fruit. A larger scar generally means fewer seeds.

✳ EGGPLANT STORAGE

Eggplant is quite perishable and will not store long. Depending on the freshness factor of the eggplant at the time of purchase, it may be refrigerated for up to 4 days (up to 7 days if you pick right from the garden). However, it is best to use them as soon as possible, preferably within a day.

Handle eggplants gingerly, as they bruise easily. If you purchase them wrapped in plastic wrap, remove the wrapper, wrap in a paper towel, and place in a perforated plastic bag before storing in the refrigerator vegetable bin. Do not store raw eggplant at temperatures less than 50 degrees F.

Cooked eggplant may be refrigerated up to 3 days (it will get mushy when reheated) or frozen up to 6 months in puree form (add a little lemon juice to discourage discoloration). It holds up fairly well in chunks in soups and stews when thawed in the refrigerator, but not as chunks on its own.

✳ EGGPLANT COOKING TIPS

- Eggplant may be steamed, baked, sauteed, boiled, microwaved, stir-fried or stuffed. They are eaten as an appetizer, main dish or as part of a melange of vegetables.
- Eggplant skin is edible. However, some find it bitter, thus some recipes require peeling.
- The flesh is very sponge-like and will soak up juices and oils.
- Once cut, eggplant flesh will begin to darken with exposure to air. A brushing of lemon juice will keep the flesh light.
- Do not use aluminum cookware with eggplant as it will cause discoloration.
- Bitterness is concentrated just under the skin, so peeling will also work on especially large eggplants.
- Eggplant may be microwaved to remove excess water. Microwave slices on high for 4 to 6 minutes, remove, cover and let stand for a minute or two. Use paper towels and press lightly to soak up the water.
- If you are baking whole eggplant, be sure to puncture the skin in several places so it does not burst.
- Add eggplant to soups and stews during the last 10 minutes to avoid overcooking.

EGGPLANT MEASURES AND EQUIVALENTS

- 1 medium eggplant = about 1 pound
- 1 medium eggplant = 4 to 6 servings
- 1 pound eggplant = 3 to 4 cups diced
- 1 serving = 1/3 pound as a side dish
- 1 serving = 1/2 to 3/4 pound as a main dish

MICROWAVE EGGPLANT

1 eggplant, about 1/2 pound
4 tablespoons olive oil
1 tablespoon minced fresh parsley
Salt

Cut the eggplant in half lengthwise. Sprinkle olive oil and a little salt over the top of each half. Place on a plate and microwave on high for 4 minutes, turning once. Sprinkle with the minced parsley. That's all.
Makes 2 servings.

EASY-TO-DO RATATOUILLE

2 Tbsp Mrs. Dash Tomato Basil Garlic Seasoning Blend
2 Tbsp olive oil
1 cup sliced onions
1 cup sliced green bell pepper
1 cup sliced red bell pepper
2 cups sliced zucchini
2 cups peeled, cubed eggplant
14.5 oz can diced tomatoes, undrained

Heat oil in a large non-stick skillet. Add onion, peppers, zucchini, and eggplant. Cook over medium heat for 8-10 minutes or until vegetables are crisp-tender. Sprinkle with Mrs. Dash Tomato Basil Garlic. Stir in tomatoes and cook over medium heat for 5 minutes or until heated thoroughly. *Makes 6 servings.*

Per Serving: Calories 89, Total Fat 5gm, Sodium 120mg

✳ BALSAMIC GRILLED VEGGIES

2 Tbsp olive oil
1 Tbsp dried or 1/4 cup chopped fresh basil
1 Tbsp balsamic vinegar
1 tsp pepper
1 large red onion, cut into 1-inch pieces
1 (8-oz.) package fresh mushrooms
1 pt. cherry tomatoes
2 medium zucchini, cut into 1-inch pieces
4 small yellow squash, cut into 1-inch pieces

Preheat grill to 350-400 degrees (medium-high heat). Stir together olive oil and next 4 ingredients in a small bowl. Rinse fennel thoroughly. Trim and discard root end of fennel bulb. Trim stalks from bulb, reserving fronds for another use. Cut bulb in half vertically, and remove core. Cut bulb into 1/2 inch thick slices. Toss fennel, onion, and mushrooms with half of olive oil mixture, and place in a grill wok or metal basket. Grill covered for 10 minutes over 350-400 degrees (medium-high heat). Toss tomatoes, zucchini, and yellow squash with remaining olive oil mixture. Add to grill wok or basket. Grill, covered with grill lid, stirring occasionally, 10 to 15 minutes or until vegetables are tender. Serve immediately. *Makes 6 servings.*

Per Serving: Calories 83, Total Fat 4.8gm, Sodium 1mg

✳ RICER RATATOUILLE

8 cups yellow squash, chopped
2 cups diced green peppers
2 Tbsp olive oil
2 Tbsp Italian seasoning
2 packets of Herb Ox No Sodium Chicken Broth
2 cans Muir Glen Organic No Salt Added Diced Tomatoes
1 can Health Valley Organic No Salt Added Tomato Soup
8 cups zucchini, chopped
2 cups diced onion

1 Tbsp minced garlic
1 Tbsp Mrs. Dash
4 cups tomatoes, chopped
8 cups cubed eggplant
1 Tbsp powdered garlic
2 packets of Splenda

Place all the above ingredients in a large pot at medium heat. Cover but leave the lid slightly elevated to allow heat to escape and prevent overcooking. Make certain to stir contents entirely and continue stirring for approximately 40 minutes. You may wish to lower the temperature to low if the ingredients are boiling. *Makes 18 cups.*

Per Serving (1 cup): Calories: 74.4, Fat: 1.8gm, Sodium: 70.7mg
Divide the recipe in half to make 9 cups, to freeze for later. Date and title before freezing. An absolutely tasty dish that can stay refrigerated up to 1 week and still taste as if you just made it. Eat it hot or cold, with rice and/or a 3 oz. serving of lean chicken, fish or beef, broiled, grilled or baked. Remember to add the calories.

RICER BROCCOLI SLAW TOMATO GARLIC RICE DISH

1 Tbsp olive oil
12oz bag Eat Smart Broccoli Slaw
2 Tbsp Vidalia Valley sweet onions and pepper
2 tsp Badia minced garlic in oil
1 packet of Herb Ox No Sodium Beef Broth
2 cups Quirch Frozen diced onions and peppers
2 cups Pictsweet Mixed Frozen Vegetables
3 cans No Salt Added Diced Tomatoes
2 tsp California sun-dried julienne cut tomatoes with oil
2 Tbsp Mrs. Dash
2 tsp onion powder
2 tsp garlic powder
5 cups cooked parboiled rice

Place 1 Tbsp olive oil in large pot on stove. Heat at medium until sizzling, then add frozen onions and peppers. Cook and stir for approximately 5 minutes. Add frozen vegetables and broccoli slaw.

Continue cooking on medium heat until the broccoli slaw is slightly limp. Add the cans of diced tomatoes with the liquid (do not drain cans) and add the rest of the ingredients. Stir thoroughly and cook over low heat for approximately 12 minutes, until desired temperature. You may eat this dish hot or cold, it's healthy, delicious and garlicky good! *Makes 15 cups.*

Per Serving (2 cups): Calories 320, Fat 2.6gm, Sodium 71mg
You may add 3 oz. cooked lean chicken, beef or fish, but make certain to add on the appropriate calories.

✳ SWEET & SOUR CABBAGE

2 cups of water
2 Tbsp Canola Oil
4 tart apples, peeled and sliced
1/4 cup Splenda brown sugar blend (packed)
8 cups shredded cabbage
6 Tbsp Vinegar
Dash of black pepper

In a large pot add water, brown sugar, vinegar, oil and pepper. Cook for 2-3 minutes, stirring occasionally on medium-low. Add the shredded cabbage, cover and cook, stirring occasionally for about 10 minutes, or until tender.

Add the apples and cook uncovered, stirring occasionally, for approximately 10 minutes, until tender. Remove from heat, let cool. *Makes 5 cups.*

Per Serving (1/2 cup): Calories 78, Fat 2.8gm, Sodium 10mg

ENTREES

RICER BEANS AND RICE LETTUCE WRAPS

Combine the following ingredients in a large bowl that holds at least 12 cups:
2 cups organic frozen corn niblets
2 cans (15oz) Eden no-sodium black beans, drained and rinsed
2 cups cooked white parboiled rice
3 cups cooked red lentils
2 red bell peppers, diced
2 yellow bell peppers, diced

Thoroughly mix the following ingredients together and then stir into the
bean and rice mixture:
6 Tbsp apple cider vinegar
4 Tbsp Badia minced garlic in oil
2 Tbsp dry chopped chives
1 head of iceberg lettuce, rinsed and dried
3 Tbsp olive oil
2 Tbsp dried cilantro
2-1/2 tsp ground cumin

Once all the items are gently and thoroughly combined, cover and
refrigerate for at least 1 hour. A serving is 1 cup. Place lettuce leaves onto a
plate and carefully spoon a tablespoon of the mixture inside. Roll or fold the
ends toward each other to meet in the middle to create your bean and rice
lettuce wrap. *Makes 12 cups.*

Per Serving (1 cup): Calories 241, Fat 3.5gm, Sodium 13mg

FISH TOFU 2GOOD2B TRUE

1 cup water
6 oz. salmon, uncooked, not frozen
6 oz. tilapia, uncooked, not frozen
3 sliced small peppers

1 cup mixed frozen vegetable

Mrs. Dash, Tumeric, Cumin, Coriander, Curry

1/2 Pkg firm tofu-cubed

1 sliced tomato

1 cup snap peas (optional)

2 cups cooked rice

2 cups lettuce

Take a large wok or frying pan and add 1 cup water. Heat on medium, then add the ingredients above. Thoroughly stir, making certain to add more water when needed, always having a bit of "broth" on the bottom of the pan. Cover and cook for approximately 15 minutes on medium or until fish is cooked completely. *Makes 8 servings.*

Per Serving: Calories 169, Fat 5gm, Sodium 23mg

✳ BAKED SALMON WITH PINEAPPLE SALSA

3 Tbsp Mrs. Dash Original Blend

1 lb. skinless salmon fillets, 1" thick, lightly sprayed with non-stick cooking spray

1/2 cup diced green peppers

1/2 cup diced red peppers

1 cup canned crushed pineapple in juice, dained with juice reserved

1 tsp finely grated fresh ginger (or use store bought spice jar of ginger)

Line a small sheet pan with non-stick aluminum foil. Arrange salmon on baking sheet. Sprinkle fillets evenly with a capful/2 Tbsp of Mrs. Dash Original Blend. Place in preheated 450 degree oven for about 10 minutes, or until fish flakes easily. Meanwhile, saute peppers in 1/4 cup reserved pineapple juice until crisp-tender. Add remaining Mrs. Dash Original Blend, pineapple and ginger. Remove from heat. Arrange salmon on serving plates topped with pineapple salsa. *Makes 4 servings.*

Per Serving (4oz fillet with 1/2 cup salsa)**:** Calories 190, Fat 6gm, Sodium 45mg

RICER CRUMBLES TOFU BROCCOLI SLAW

10 oz package of Marjon Tofu Crumbles
2 cups kale, packaged
2 cups cooked rice
2 cups mixed frozen vegetables
Dash of Turmeric, Curry, and Cumin
1 cup water (season with Herb Ox Sodium Free Chicken or Beef Bouillon if desired)
12 oz. bag of broccoli slaw
15 oz. can of diced tomatoes, no salt, drained
1 cup sliced fresh mushrooms
2 Tbsp Albertos Sweet Jalapeño Relish (optional - you may substitute this ingredient with 1 Tbsp of apple cider vinegar, 1 packet of Splenda Sweetener, 1 Tbsp of minced onions (dehydrated from spice bottle) OR 1/4 cups diced raw onions, and add all together in a cup, stir well, add to food as you begin to cook.)

Place water in large pot or pan at medium heat and bring to a boil (add Herb Ox bouillon if desired). Add the kale, mixed frozen vegetables, broccoli slaw, diced tomatoes, sliced fresh mushrooms and rice, one ingredient at a time. Stir. Add the spices. Add more water if necessary (there should always be a small amount of water at the bottom of the pan/pot so that it doesn't stick to the pan). Cook for approximately 15 minutes, covered, stirring often until hot and slightly bubbly. *Makes 4 servings.*

Per Serving: Calories 158, Fat 3.1gm, Sodium 60mg

RICER SAUCY EGGPLANT CRUMBLE RAGOUT

2 Tbsp virgin Olive Oil
2 medium eggplants, peeled, cubed
4 10 oz. pkgs Marjon Tofu Crumbles
1 10 oz. pkg fresh matchstick carrots
1 14.5 oz can Muir Glen organic diced tomatoes, no salt added
1 Tbsp Badia minced garlic in oil

8 oz. pkg Nasoya organic cubed tofu
12 oz. pkg fresh sliced mushrooms
12 oz. pkg fresh broccoli slaw
15-1/2 oz. jar low sodium spaghetti sauce, no sugar/sodium added

Place olive oil in a large pot, heat, add mushrooms and eggplant cubes, and stir gently until slightly softened. Add the remaining ingredients, stir gently and cook until desired temperature. Add whatever other seasonings you prefer, i.e. oregano, dill, Mrs. Dash, garlic, hot pepper, turmeric. Place on serving of rice, baked potato, or rice noodles; you must add the calories for the serving of the starch product chosen. *Makes 26 cups.*

Per Serving (1 cup): Calories 82, Fat 4gm, Sodium 25mg

✳ CHICKEN AND VEGGIE KABOBS

3/4 cup Mrs. Dash Lemon Herb Peppercorn Marinade
1 lb boneless, skinless, chicken breast, cut into 1 inch cubes
12 cherry tomatoes
2 small zucchini, cut into 12 1/2 inch pieces
2 medium red onions, cut into eighths
4 long skewers

Marinate chicken cubes in Mrs. Dash Lemon Herb Peppercorn Marinade for 10 minutes. Thread skewers with chicken and alternate with vegetables. Preheat grill to medium high and grill kabobs for 3 minutes, then turn and grill for another 3 minutes or until done. For extra flavor, brush kabobs with more marinade. *Makes 4 servings.*

Per Serving (1 Kabob): Calories 180, Total Fat 2gm, Sodium 86mg

✳ RICER KASHA CHILI

28 oz No Salt Diced Tomatoes
5 packets of Herb Ox No Salt Beef Broth
5 cups of water
1 15 oz can Eden Organic Kidney Beans, No Salt Added, drained

1 Tbsp chili powder
1 tsp paprika
2 Tbsp Mrs. Dash Original Blend
1 Tbsp minced onion
2 Tbsp Heinz No Salt Ketchup
1 tsp garlic powder
1 tsp cumin
1/2 tsp black coarse ground pepper
1 tsp oregano
1 13oz box Wolff's Kasha

In a large skillet, add all ingredients EXCEPT KASHA. Bring to a gentle boil. Add the box of kasha, stir, cover and cook for approximately 10 minutes on low heat or simmer. Make certain it is not continuously boiling, so lower the heat and keep covered. Continue cooking until the kasha is tender, for approximately another 5 minutes. *Makes 11 cups.*

Per Serving (1 cup): Calories 174, Fat .7gm, Sodium 25mg

SALAD

TANGY CUCUMBER RICER SALAD
1 tsp Mrs. Dash Garlic & Herb Seasoning Blend
3/8 cup apple cider vinegar*
3 large cucumbers finely chopped or thinly sliced
16 oz. container Stonyfield OIKOS 0% fat Organic Greek Yogurt-Plain (or use FAGE Greek Yogurt)
1/2 tsp Mrs. Dash Lemon Pepper Seasoning Blend*
2 packets of Splenda
1 Vadalia onion (sweet) minced or finely chopped
2 cups cooked and cooled/cold parboiled rice (or other)

Combine the Mrs. Dash Garlic and Herb and Lemon Pepper seasonings in a large glass or plastic bowl** along with the apple cider vinegar and Splenda.

Mix thoroughly. Fold in the Greek Yogurt and mix well. At this point you may wish to take a very large Ziploc bag to blend all the ingredients together or continue mixing in your large bowl. Add the cucumbers, onions and cooked cooled/cold rice. Gently stir (or if in a bag turn the bag over and over—make certain it is absolutely zipped closed!) to coat all the food. Store in the refrigerator for approximately 2 hours to allow the flavors to meld. *Makes 10 servings.*

*This is a tangy/spicy dish. If you wish, you can use less vinegar and 1/4 tsp of the lemon pepper seasoning.

** Avoid using aluminum products when cooking with yogurt (bowls, pots, utensils) as the acidity of yogurt can react negatively with aluminum.

Per Serving (1 cup): Calories 200, Fat .3gm, Sugar 3.6g, Sodium 23mg

✱ CARROT SALAD

2 Tbsp Mrs. Dash Onion and Herb Seasoning Blend
1 lb carrots, grated
1/2 cup raisins
1/2 cup walnuts, chopped
1 cup yogurt with fruit, low-fat pineapple or lemon
1 Tbsp brown sugar

Toss grated carrots, raisins, and walnuts. Mix together yogurt, Mrs. Dash Onion and Herb and brown sugar. Add to carrot mixture and mix well. Cover and refrigerate. *Makes 6 servings.*

Per Serving (5 oz): Calories 166, Calories from Fat 43%, Total Fat 8gm, Saturated Fat 1gm, Unsaturated Fat 6gm, Trans Fat 0gm

✱ EDAMAME SUCCOTASH SALAD

2 Tbsp extra-virgin olive oil
1 medium onion, chopped
1 bag (16oz) shelled edamame (soybeans), thawed

1 bag (16oz) thawed corn kernels
2 large ripe plum tomatoes, diced
1/4 tsp ground black pepper
1/4 cup minced fresh chives or basil

Heat oil in a 4-quart saucepan over medium heat. Add onion and cook, stirring often, until softened but not browned, 4-5 minutes. Add the edamame and corn, turning often, until heated through, about 7 minutes. Stir in the tomato and pepper. Let cool, then chill if being used later. When ready to serve, stir in the minced fresh chives or basil.

Makes 10 servings, 5 cups.

Per Serving (1/2 cup): Calories 125, Fat 5gm, Sodium 18.5mg

MIDDLE EASTERN RICE SALAD

3 Tbsp olive oil
1 thinly sliced sweet onion
6 cups cooked brown rice
2 - 15oz cans Edan Organic no salt added garbanzo beans (chick peas)
1 tsp ground pepper
1 cup california chopped dates (sunsweet)
1 tsp ground cumin
1/2 cup chopped fresh parsley
1/2 cup chopped fresh mint

In a large pan, add 3 Tbsp olive oil and heat until slight sizzle is heard. Add the thinly sliced sweet onion and cook until slightly browned, approximately 6 minutes. Remove from heat. Add the remaining ingredients. Toss well. Serve warm, room temperature or cold, depending on preference. This dish would be great on the side or as part of a main dish with shredded lettuce, tomatoes, cucumbers, mushrooms, or green and red peppers…use your imagination, BUT always remember to add the calories.

Makes 12 cups.

Per Serving (1 cup): Calories 313, Fat 4gm, Sodium 18.4mg

DESERTS

✳ CINNAMON PEACH COBBLER
6 peaches
1/2 cup oatmeal
2 tsp cinnamon
1/2 tsp allspice

Preheat oven to 375. Peel and seed the peaches, then cut so you have about 6 pieces per peach. In a 2" pan, combine peaches, cinnamon and allspice and mix lightly. Cover and bake for 20 minutes, stirring once. Mix in uncooked oatmeal, cover and bake another 5 minutes. *Makes 4 servings.*

Per Serving: Calories 106, Calories from fat 6%, Fat 1gm, Sodium 1mg

✳ BAKED PINEAPPLE-BLUEBERRY COBBLER
1 cup pineapple chunks (fresh or canned, preferably no syrup)
1 1/2 cup blueberries (fresh or frozen)
1 cup dry oatmeal
1/2 cup pineapple juice
1 tsp vanilla
1 tsp cinnamon

Preheat oven to 350 degrees. Spoon pineapple into bottom of baking dish. Add oatmeal on top of pineapple. Add blueberries on top of oatmeal. Mix juice, vanilla, and cinnamon in bowl. Pour over blueberries. Bake uncovered for 20-25 minutes. The cobbler is done when oatmeal has thickened and browned and some blueberries have risen to the top. Serve warm. Leftovers can be stored in the refrigerator for 1-2 days. *Makes 8 servings.*

Per Serving (1/2 cup): Calories 70, Fat 1gm, Saturated Fat 0gm, Fiber 2g, Sodium 1mg

RICER DESSERT SMORES

1 Bible Bread Cracker (Chamberlain's) -OR- 3 GILDA no salt/sugar crackers
1 tsp Walden Farms, Calorie Free, Creamy Peanut Spread (Chamberlain's)
1 Tbsp Walden Farms Marshmallow Dip (Chamberlain's)
1 Tbsp Walden Farms Caramel or Chocolate Dip (Chamberlain's)

Take the Bible Bread –OR- GILDA crackers (no salt/no sugar) and evenly
spread the Peanut Spread, followed by the Marshmallow Dip,
then a layer of the Caramel or Chocolate Dip. ENJOY! Serve with some
fresh fruit for a simply fabulous dessert. *Makes 1 cracker of bible bread or 2
gilda no salt/no sugar crackers*

Per Serving: Calories 45, Fat 0gm, Sodium 43mg

QUICK APPLE CRISP DESSERT

Microwave chopped apples topped with sprinkled cinnamon. Serve with a
sprinkle of rolled oats and Seelect Sodium Free Maple Syrup or Splenda.

PUMPKIN PIE COTTAGE CHEESE AND RAISINS

Almost as good as pumpkin pie—give it a try!
1/2 cup canned Organic Pumpkin Pie Mix*
1/2 cup cottage cheese
2 tsp of raisins
pinch of cinnamon

Mix cottage cheese and pumpkin pie. Mix thoroughly. Add cinnamon and
raisins. Serve with sliced apples or other fruits. Also delicious served on
Gilda crackers, Melba Toast or other permitted crackers.

*If you use the Organic Plain Pumpkin Pie, you may use Pumpkin Pie Spice
(found in most stores in a jar) or make your own. You may wish to add 2
tsp. Walden Farms Maple Pancake Syrup or 1 packet of Splenda or Stevia if
you desire a sweeter taste. If you use 1 tsp. of honey, make certain to add 20
more calories. **Per Serving (3/4 cup):** Calories 210, Fat 1.5gm, Sodium 65mg

Pumpkin Pie Spice:

If pumpkin pie spice isn't available or you wish to make your own mixture: use 1/2 tsp of cinnamon, 1/4 tsp of ginger and 1/8 tsp of allspice to stand in for 1 tsp of the blend. Some folks add cloves instead of allspice. Most commercial brands, such as McCormick's, have four ingredients: cinnamon, ginger, nutmeg and allspice.

Other uses for canned pumpkin pie:
- Add 1-2 Tbsp raisins to 1/2 cup rice with a dash of cinnamon
- Add to Oatmeal
- Use as a dip for sliced apples
- Stir into 1/2 cup Greek Yogurt
- Substitute canned pumpkin (or applesauce) for eggs or oil in some baked recipes

DRESSINGS, SAUCES AND RELISHES

✳ RICER SALSA BASE

To 1/2 cup no salt tomato sauce, add:
2 Tbsp of each of the following diced or finely chopped:
cucumber, onions, green pepper, tomato (may be found at your local grocery store in small containers already prepared)
Add Mrs. Dash if desired.

✳ LOW SODIUM SOY SAUCE

2 Tbsp sodium free beef bouillon (use the Herb Ox)
2 tsp red wine vinegar
1 tsp molasses
1/8 tsp ground ginger
Dash of black pepper and garlic powder
3/4 cup water

In a small saucepan, combine and boil gently uncovered about 5 minutes or until mixture is reduced to 1/2 cup. Store in the refrigerator. Stir before using. *Makes 8 servings.*

Per Serving (1 Tbsp): Calories 10, Fat 0gm, Sodium 5mg

RICE DIET TOMATO SAUCE

For each serving, use 2 ripe, peeled tomatoes, 1/4 whole green pepper cut into pieces, and 1/4 medium onion, diced. Boil together over medium heat until onions and green pepper are soft. Add a little water if you desire a thinner sauce. If you wish to make the sauce thicker, continue boiling until it thickens.

RICE DIET SALAD DRESSING

Puree the following in a blender or food processor: 1 ripe peeled tomato, 1 small diced onion, the juice of 1 lemon, 1/2 cup cooked white rice, 1 packet of sodium-free sweetener, 1/4 cup mineral oil. This works well on salads or over baked potatoes.

CRANBERRY-APPLE-PINEAPPLE NO SUGAR RELISH

12-ounce bag fresh cranberries, rinsed
2 6-ounce bags organic sliced apples
1 can Geisha crushed pineapple in natural juice, drained
6 Tbsp Seelect Maple Pancake Syrup
3 packets of Splenda
1/2 tsp of cinnamon
1/4 tsp lemon juice (optional)

In a food processor with a metal knife blade, PULSE some of the cranberries and apple slices with the cinnamon, 3 packets Splenda and some of the Seelect Syrup. Place mixture into a large container that can hold 5-1/4 cups. Add the can of drained crushed pineapple, lemon juice if desired, and stir repeatedly until thoroughly mixed. Adjust according to taste, i.e. add more lemon juice or sweetener. Place covered container into the refrigerator for several hours. Eat plain or on permitted crackers. YUM! *5 1/4 cups makes 21 servings; 1/4 cup makes 1 serving.*

Per Serving (1/4 cup): Calories 30, Fat 0gm, Sodium .2mg

✳ RICER SALSA THAT'LL KNOCK YOUR SOCKS OFF!

1 can Muir Glen Organic No Salt Added Diced Tomatoes, 14.5 oz
1 Tbsp lime juice + 1 Tbsp lemon juice
1/4 tsp minced garlic (powder)
1 Tbsp Mrs. Dash
1 Tbsp chopped minced onions (dehydrated)
2 Tbsp parsley (dehydrated)
2 Tbsp chopped green peppers

Stir all ingredients together in a bowl and refrigerate for several hours. Serve with veggies. Guilt-free snacking! *1 1/2 cups makes 6 servings; 1/4 cup makes 1 serving.*

Per Serving (1/4 cup): Calories 16, Fat 0gm, Sodium 8mg

✳ SPICY PINEAPPLE SAUCE FOR RICE

2 (20 oz) cans crushed pineapple in pineapple juice
2 tsp ground ginger
2 Tbsp cornstarch
1-1/2 cups pure squeezed OJ
3/4 cup Quirch frozen diced onions and peppers
4 Tbsp SEELECT maple syrup OR 100% pure maple syrup with the lowest calories/sodium.

You may wish to add the following items, making certain to add the calories: Cooked rice; tofu and/or black beans; cooked lean chicken, beef or fish.

In a bowl, add the 2 cans of crushed pineapple with the juice, ginger and cornstarch and mix well. In a pot, place the orange juice and maple syrup over a medium heat and cook for approximately 7 minutes while stirring. Mix in the pineapple mixture, onions and peppers. At this point if you wish to add any of the other ingredients (tofu, beans, cooked chicken, beef or fish), you may do so. Continue cooking over a medium heat for approximately 20 minutes, stirring periodically, making certain not to allow the sauce to stick to the bottom of the pot. Keep the heat distributed and enable the sauce to thicken.

Per Serving (1/2 cup): Calories 82, Fat 0gm, Sodium 1mg

BALSAMIC GLAZED VEGGIES AS CONDIMENT OR TOPPING

3 Tbsp Smart Balance whipped low sodium spread
3 Tbsp balsamic vinegar
1-8 oz container chopped green peppers
2-14.5 oz cans no salt added diced tomatos (do not drain, use all liquid)
1-14.5 oz package frozen seasoning blend (chopped onions, peppers, celery, parsley)
3 Tbsp Splenda brown sugar blend
2 tsp chopped garlic in jar
1/4 cup dry oatmeal

In a pot that can hold 6 cups, melt Smart Balance, Splenda brown sugar, balsamic vinegar and garlic until blended; add the rest of the ingredients. Cook on high, stirring until the mixture is slightly thickened. Remove from heat. Serve hot or cold. This can be eaten as a condiment for Ricer-recommended crackers, with raw veggies or placed on rice, baked potato, and more. Just make certain to add the calories of whatever other product you are eating with this. *Makes 6 cups.*

Per Serving (1/4 cup): Calories 39, Fat 1gm, Sodium 18mg, Sugar 4g

YOGURT SUBSTITUTION GUIDE (1 TBSP)

	Calories	Total Fat (g)	Protein (g)	Calcium
Regular Mayonnaise	96	11		
Light Mayonnaise	45	4		
Regular Sour Cream	31	3		2%
Light Sour Cream	19	1	< 1	
Regular Cream Cheese	51	5		1%
Light Cream Cheese	35	2.5		2%
Heavy Cream	51	5.5		1%
Light Cream	29	3		1%
Half n' Half	20	1.5		2%
Butter (unsalted)	102	11.5		
Margarine	54	6		
Vegetable Oil	121	13.5		
Fat Free Plain Yogurt	7		< 1	3%
Low Fat Plain Yogurt	8	< 0.5	< 1	3%
Whole Milk Plain Yogurt	11	0.5	< 1	3%
Oikos Plain Greek Yogurt	8		2	2%
Oikos Vanilla Greek Yogurt	10		2	2%

YOGURT SUBSTITUTION GUIDE (1/2 CUP)

	Calories	Total Fat (g)	Protein (g)	Calcium
Regular Mayonnaise	770	88		
Light Mayonnaise	360	33		
Regular Sour Cream	246	24		14%
Light Sour Cream	153	10	5	3%
Regular Cream Cheese	405	40.5		10%

YOGURT SUBSTITUTION GUIDE (1/2 CUP) CONTINUED

	Calories	Total Fat (g)	Protein (g)	Calcium
Light Cream Cheese	277	21		14%
Heavy Cream	411	44		8%
Light Cream	234	23		12%
Half n' Half	158	14		13%
Butter (unsalted)	814	92		3%
Margarine	428	48		1%
Vegetable Oil	964	109		
Fat Free Plain Yogurt	55		6	20%
Low Fat Plain Yogurt	60	1	5	20%
Whole Milk Plain Yogurt	90	4.5	5	20%
Oikos Plain Greek Yogurt	60		12	15%
Oikos Vanilla Greek Yogurt	80		11	13%

SIDE DISHES

SPANISH RICE

Add 1 cup Rice Diet Tomato Sauce to 1 cup cooked white rice. Cook over medium heat until most of the liquid evaporates and the mixture is thickened. Fresh mushrooms may be added, if you wish. Makes 2 servings.

RICER RICE STUFFING, A NEW TRADITION

1 cup cooked rice
1 Tbsp minced onions (dehydrated)
1 tsp crumbled Rosemary
1 packet of Herb Ox sodium free broth
1/2 cup no salt canned mushrooms Pennsylvania Dutch, drained
1 Tbsp Mrs. Dash
3 GILDA crackers
1/2 cup hot water

Break up the GILDA crackers (place in a zip lock bag and pound on it). Mix the Herb Ox broth to 1/2 cup hot water and add the crushed crackers. Combine well, let the broth be absorbed by the crackers, then mix all the ingredients together. Microwave on HIGH for 3-1/2 minutes...it's better than the real thing. Truly a great stuffing, just don't stuff yourself with it! *1 1/2 cups makes 3 servings; 1/2 cup makes 1 serving.*

Per Serving (1/2 cup): Calories 62, Fat .7gm, Sodium 8mg

✳ PASTA ALFREDO WITH EDAMAME, TOMATOES AND PEPPERS

16oz package Tinkyada Brown Rice Pasta Fusilli
1/2 cup frozen Edamame, shelled
6 Tbsp Walden Farms Alfredo Sauce, calorie free
14.5 oz can no salt added diced tomatoes, drained
5 cups water
1/4 cup frozen diced green peppers
1 Tbsp Galaxy Nutritional Foods Veggie Grated Topping

Place 5 cups water in 4 or 5 quart pot. Place on stove at high temperature. Add the Edamame and green pepper. Bring to a boil. Add the entire package of Rice Pasta Fusilli, stir, boil for 1-2 minutes. Remove from the heat and let sit covered for 12 minutes. Drain. Add drained can of tomatoes, alfredo sauce and grated cheese. Stir gently. *Makes 10 cups.*

Per Serving (1 cup): Calories 194, Fat 2.2gm, Sodium 37mg

✳ RICER EXTRA SPICY RICE

2 cups cooked rice (brown, white, basmati or jasmine, parboiled)
1 chopped onion
2 packets of Herb Ox No Sodium Chicken Broth (to sprinkle onto rice, don't dilute in water)
2 tsp Mrs. Dash Extra Spicy Seasoning Blend
2 Tbsp chopped parsley
2 Tbsp Smart Balance Margarine

Add all ingredients together; cook in microwave on high for 8 minutes or until desired temperature.

Per Serving (1/2 cup): Calories 180, Fat 3.5gm, Sodium 15mg

CRISP APPLE SLICES WITH PEANUT BUTTER YOGURT DIP
16oz container Chobani non-fat greek vanilla yogurt
1 Tbsp honey
1 tsp cinnamon
6 Tbsp low-sodium Better 'n Peanut Butter

Mix all ingredients together. Use immediately or refrigerate until ready for use. For a smoother consistency, gradually add 1 Tbsp warm water and stir. You may choose not to add the peanut butter and just have the apples with the yogurt as a dip. *Makes 18oz container of dip.*

Per Serving (2 Tbsp): Calories 35, Fat .3gm, Sodium 24mg
Remember to add the calories of the apple slices (1 apple = 12 slices), 90 calories.

THREE BEAN RICE SIDE SALAD
8 cups cooked, cold temperature Uncle Ben's 7 Grains Medley
15oz can Eden Organic Black Beans, no salt added
15oz can Eden Organic Garbanzo Beans, no salt added
1 cup cooked/cooled frozen shelled edamame
1/4 cup olive oil
1/4 cup balsamic vinegar
1/2 Tbsp Mrs. Dash seasonings
1/8 tsp black pepper
1/8 tsp garlic powder (or less)
1/2 Tbsp minced onion

Place cooked rice into a large bowl or large plastic bag. Add the remainder of all ingredients, mix thoroughly. *Makes 11 cups.*

Per Serving (1 cup): Calories 250, Fat 15gm, Sodium 16mg

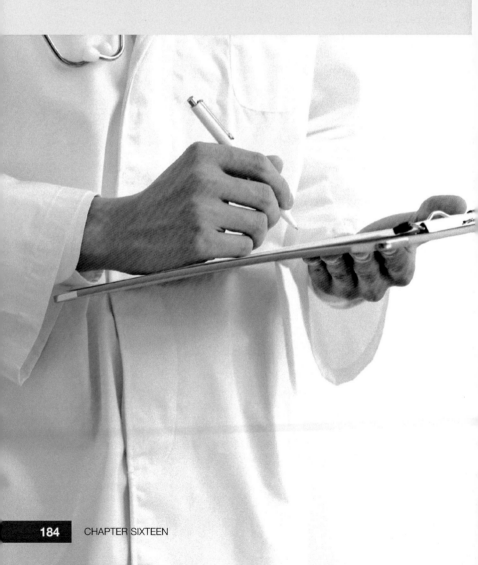

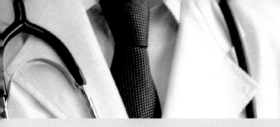

CHAPTER SIXTEEN
RICE DIET CONTRACT AND JOURNAL

YOUR RICE DIET CONTRACT AND JOURNAL ARE NOT FRIVOLOUS "FEEL GOOD" EXERCISES. They are key instruments in pledging and fulfilling your commitment to defeating obesity and attaining your ideal weight.

Your Rice Diet contract confirms in writing your commitment to changing your life and improving your health. Please read and sign this document as you would any contract, then:

- Keep one signed copy for ready reference
- Give a signed copy of your contract to your doctor and anyone else you wish to share it with (family, friends, fellow dieters, etc.)

While your contract has no legal power per se, it binds you spiritually and emotionally to your commitment to good health. Take it seriously, respect its power, and embrace it as an affirmation of your unshakable determination to be healthy and happy!

Your Rice Diet journal will help you succeed with your diet by allowing you to gain insight into your eating behavior and the emotional states that cause them. Fill in your journal on a daily basis, recording everything you eat and drink, your exercising for the day, and your feelings as they relate to your emotional outlook.

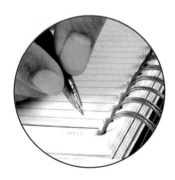

"EAT, WRITE, REFLECT, REDIRECT"

Your Rice Diet journal is an amazingly power instrument of change, so use it!

CONTRACT TO COMMIT TO LIVING A NEW LIFESTYLE, A HEALTHY LIFESTYLE

This contract is comprised of goals that you wish to attain. Commit to working toward these goals on a daily basis. Review this page when you make your daily entries in your journal. The blanks that you fill in will enable you to fill in the blanks toward a better understanding of yourself, your behavior, your actions, why you do the things you do and how to avoid doing them. You will gain insight into how to become a healthier you, mentally, physically and emotionally.

I, _____, COMMIT to making a change in my lifestyle, toward becoming a healthier person. I realize that this will not happen overnight. I realize that my actions are integral to my success or failure to reach the goals I wish to achieve. If I wish to succeed, I will need to focus on DOING the following toward my success:

_____ Become more active

_____ Weigh myself on a daily basis

_____ Get a healthier attitude about myself, letting my self-esteem rise

_____ Energize myself

_____ All of the above. DO IT.

I will commit to staying on track, to enable change to occur. I will motivate myself to stick to everything that is required to enable a successful outcome.

One way I can motivate myself is to keep this goal in mind:

_____

(example: school or family reunion; fitting into your favorite clothing)

Possible roadblocks and how I will overcome them:

_____

_____

_____

(example: lunching with friends and ordering what they order; snacks sitting around at work; 2 for 1 specials at the supermarket-such as cookies, donuts and other no-no's; watching television with the 'need' to eat along with watching the program.)

These are the commitments I will make:

_____ I want to aspire to be healthy
_____ I want to live a healthier lifestyle
_____ I want to get healthy and stay healthy
_____ I will not make any more excuses
_____ I will do what I need to do to reach my goals
_____ I will follow the Rice Diet, because it is the
right diet...for me.

_____

Signature

_____

Date

MY RICE DIET AND EXERCISE JOURNAL

DAY _____   DATE _____

WATER: 8 oz. glasses of water consumed today:

___ ___ ___ ___ ___ ___ ___ ___ ___

Time/Meal	Hunger	Food/Beverage/Snacks	Situation/Feelings
	1-not hungry *5-very hungry*	*(rice cake, fruit, diet drink, etc.)* *INDICATE AMOUNTS, LIKES,* *DISLIKES, ANY PREFERENCES*	*before and after eating*
Breakfast			
Lunch			
Dinner			

WALKS:	DISTANCE	TIME	STEPS	CALORIES
#1				
#2				

OTHER EXERCISE:

NOTES: (Thoughts, Feelings, Successes and Lessons Learned Today)

*Visit **www.RiceDietCF.com** to download these and other useful forms.*

KEEP A JOURNAL OR DIARY:

Below are some ideas you may wish to include:

NOTES/REMINDERS/THINGS TO DO TODAY

_____

_____

_____

_____

WHAT I LEARNED FROM YESTERDAY_____

_____

_____

WHAT I WOULD DO DIFFERENTLY TOMORROW _____

_____

_____

WHAT I AM MOST PROUD OF _____

_____

_____

Enjoy life; it is not a dress rehearsal. Always remember—live your life, not your age. Treat others the way you would wish to be treated. Yesterday is history, tomorrow is a mystery, and today is a gift—that is why they call it the "present!" ALL THINGS ARE POSSIBLE. We're more alike than we are different. "Love like you've never been hurt; dance like no one's watching! Live like it's heaven on earth. Make each day better than the day before. Be happy, be gentle to yourself, and believe in yourself." DO IT!

RICE DIET OF CENTRAL FLORIDA

NAME _____

Day	Date	BP	Weight	BLOOD SUGAR AM	PM	Waist	COMMENTS
1							
2							
3							
4							
5							
6							
7							
8							
9							
10							
11							
12							
13							
14							
15							
16							
17							
18							
19							
20							
21							
22							
23							
24							
25							
26							
27							
28							

*Visit **www.RiceDietCF.com** to download these and other useful forms.*

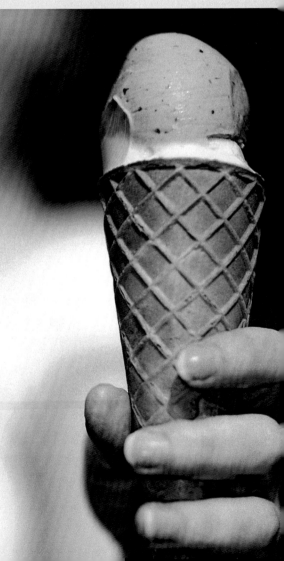

CHAPTER SEVENTEEN
PREVENTING EMOTIONAL EATING AND CHEATING

EMOTIONAL EATING AND CHEATING ON YOUR DIET ARE PERHAPS THE TWO BIGGEST CHALLENGES FACING A RICER. This chapter will help you understand the causes and symptoms of these behaviors, and show you how to resolve them without falling off your diet.

We have included an Emotional Eating Worksheet to help you pinpoint the emotional triggers that can lead you to eat unhealthily. You may fill in this worksheet or download a template at *www. ricedietcf.com*. Please read this chapter carefully and take our tips and suggestions to heart. They can greatly increase your ability to successfully maintain your diet.

ARE YOU EATING YOUR EMOTIONS?

People eat for many different reasons. True hunger is the healthiest reason to eat. Learning to eat in response to physical cues, such as hunger pangs, is a very important skill for managing calorie intake. Unfortunately, emotions, both positive and negative, can trigger the desire to eat for many people. This is called psychological hunger. Eating in response to psychological hunger can be difficult to distinguish from the hunger associated with the body's need for food. You can use a Food Log to help you pay attention to how you're feeling when you eat, and what situations trigger you to eat when you're not physically hungry.

WHY ARE PEOPLE EMOTIONAL EATERS?

Food is a mood manager for different reasons. For some people, it is a way to escape from uncomfortable emotions, such as stress, anger, or boredom. Food and eating can also enhance positive feelings, such as celebration and relaxation. Food provides comfort during times of sadness and people often describe food as soothing, numbing, or distracting. Some people even describe food as a trusted and familiar friend. You may already be aware of certain emotions that influence how you eat.

DO THESE EMOTIONS AFFECT YOUR FOOD CHOICES AND EATING PATTERNS?

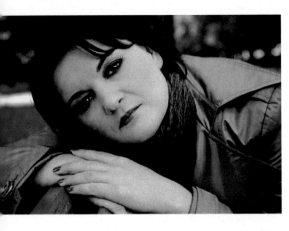

- Loneliness
- Depression
- Stress
- Anger
- Sadness
- Happiness
- Fatigue
- Anxiety
- Boredom
- Excitement
- Feeling of guilt

THE CYCLE OF EMOTIONAL EATING

Completely abandon efforts, tell yourself you don't care and deserve to have some pleasure in life, feelings of hopelessness

Triggering event or situation: weight gain, eating a "forbidden" food, an upsetting comment from someone

Eat more, binge eat, or temporarily abandon healthy eating efforts

Experience uncomfortable emotions and thoughts: negative feelings, stress, lack of control

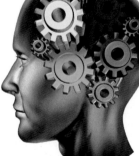

Desire to feel better: need for comfort, escape, or control

Desire to feel better: need for comfort, escape, or control

Feelings of guilt, failure, or disappointment: feeling that you blew it or lost control, ate "forbidden" foods

Eat to feel better: often includes eating "comfort foods" and a sense of escape or detachment while eating

Break the cycle! See tips for preventing emotional eating later in this chapter.

SIGNS AND SYMPTOMS OF STRESS

How do you know if you are suffering from stress? Below is a list of signs and symptoms of stress. If you are experiencing two or more symptoms from the groups below, then chances are you are over stressed.

Physical Signs of Stress

Biting your nails or grinding your teeth
Hunching your shoulders
Picking your skin
Tapping your fingers or your feet, jiggling your knees
Fiddling with your hair

Emotional Signs of Stress

Anxiety/Depression/Anger
Feelings of helplessness
Feeling impatient/restless
Feeling out of control
Losing your sense of humor
Feeling overwhelmed

Behavioral Signs of Stress

Disturbed sleep
Emotional outbursts
Aggression
Trying to do lots of things at once and not finishing any of them
Overreacting
Talking too fast and/or too loud
Frequently not hearing what people say to you

All of these stress symptoms are felt by everyone from time to time. However, if you start experiencing several of these symptoms more frequently, you need to take action to reduce your stress before it gets out of control.

GETTING TO KNOW YOUR EATING BEHAVIOR

Eating Habits - Preliminary approach to understanding
You may not actually be physically hungry. You may be stressed, tired, or bored, but you decide to eat. While eating...

1. Do you usually eat quickly? _____ Yes _____ No
2. Do you taste the food? _____ Yes _____ No
3. Are you thinking about the food? _____ Yes _____ No
4. How are you feeling?

_____ excited _____stressed _____ numb
_____ the need to clean your plate _____ angry
_____ happy _____ anxious _____ guilty

The Triggers
What were you doing before you decided to eat?

_____ watching TV
_____ just arrived home from work
_____ at a meeting at work
_____ passed by a bakery/grocery store
_____ in the break room at work
_____ saw someone else eating
_____ bored
_____ tired
_____ making a meal
_____ drove by fast food
_____ saw a vending machine
_____ preparing a snack for
someone else
_____ opened the refrigerator
_____ opened a cabinet where
you store food/snacks

Begin thinking about how to avoid the triggers

When you arrive home from work, you can eat OR

_____

_____

You drive home every day passing the same fast food restaurant that you always stop at. What can you do to change this behavior?

_____

_____

You see food in the break room at work every day. What can you do?

_____

_____

Someone offers to share a donut with you, you...

_____

_____

Snacks are available for staff meetings, i.e., chips, pretzels, salted nuts, etc. What are some options?

_____

_____

You begin eating your meal and feel that as soon as you get started, you're almost finished. What are some things you can do to take more time to eat your meal and not eat like a boa?

_____

_____

You're not physically hungry (your stomach isn't growling, you've eaten only hours ago), but you're thinking about the day, the exam, the things you need to get done before the next day...and the "stuff" that causes anxiety, stress, etc. You head toward the "comfort zone" for a pick me up. You have choices. If you choose to eat, what can you have that won't make you have regrets?

_____

_____

You receive a phone call from a friend who just arrived in town. You decide to meet for lunch. You'll be meeting in an hour, not far from where you are. You decide to meet at a mutually convenient location, such as Outback Steakhouse. You're looking forward to the lunch date, but what can you do in advance regarding your meal?

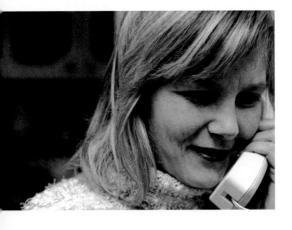

_____

_____

_____

_____

You're involved in a project that requires you to participate with packaging food at a local food Bank. You'll be there most of the day, working alongside your co-workers. Lunch is being supplied by your company. How can you prepare for this day?

_____

_____

You're dining out. You greet the server, who can make this a wonderful dining experience by accommodating your health concern requests. You order your meal, but it arrives exactly the way it was described on the menu, not the way you ordered it. You tell the server, who is very apologetic, but waiting to hear what you wish to do. What can you do?

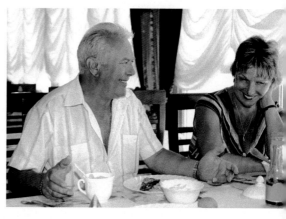

_____

_____

_____

You planned on going for a walk. You have your pedometer on, and you're ready to go. All of a sudden it begins raining. You're in the kitchen thinking about what you should do. What can you do?

_____

_____

_____

If there was a hidden camera in your house, wherever you keep food, what would you be caught eating (before or after mealtime)?

_____

_____

When you find yourself with nothing to do, what are some non-food things you can do?

_____

_____

_____

_____

_____

_____

When you were a kid, scored for the team and won the game, had a role in the school play, or received high grades in your classes, how was this handled/acknowledged by your family?

_____

_____

When you hear the word "food," what associations do you make? What comes to mind?

_____

_____

Do you to want to eat even when you're not hungry? Can you think about some of the emotions you were experiencing that triggered you to eat?

_____

_____

_____

Do you have any specific rituals when preparing or eating your food? For instance, cutting it up into small pieces, keeping food products separate from one another?

_____

_____

It's 11 AM and you're starting to get hungry. What do you do before having lunch?

_____

_____

It's been a pretty stressful day. What do you typically do to deal with the stress?

_____

_____

How do you celebrate a great accomplishment, task, purchase?

_____

_____

_____

_____

_____

_____

_____

_____

_____

TIPS FOR PREVENTING EMOTIONAL EATING AND CHEATING

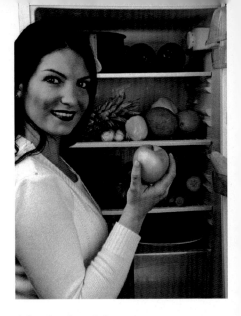

- Remember, your mind controls your thoughts. So take your mind off food and think about other things.
- We all experience stress, anxiety, fear and other negative emotions, but eating DOES NOT resolve them.
- Even Superman had a weakness—kryptonite. So he avoided it. Likewise, avoid food when it becomes your weakness.
- A snack can be unhealthy—or healthy. You have a choice, so make the right one!
- Wrong choice snacks: chips, cookies, candy bars, etc.
- Right choice snacks: Fruits, vegetables, plain yogurt with spices and unsalted nuts, etc.
- Organize your kitchen so you have healthy snacks easily in reach when you want them.
- Food high in sodium, fat and sugar cause you to want to eat more. Read the labels and avoid such foods.
- After a meal, brush your teeth with a minty toothpaste or rinse your mouth with a clean-tasting mouthwash; this can help you avoid post-meal snacking.
- Chew a piece of minty, sugar free gum to ward off a snack attack.
- "Cook large/Store small"—Cook more than a meal's worth of food and store leftovers for a healthy snack or your next meal.
- Make your own on-the-go snacks, and store in small plastic bags to take with you.

- Try drinking two full glasses of water before each meal.
- Fiber is filling—fruits, vegetables, barley, oatmeal and mushrooms are high-fiber foods that also act as appetite suppressants.
- Be mindful of your eating. Eat slowly to savor and enjoy your food.
- Use healthy substitutes whenever possible, such as:
    - PAM spray or water in a pan instead of fat for sautéing
    - Greek yogurt (such as Gage or Oikos Low Sodium type) instead of sour cream
    - Applesauce instead of butter in baked recipes
    - Salt-free cottage cheese in place of other cottage cheeses (for snacking) or ricotta cheese (for recipes)
    - Tofu crumbles instead of ground beef
    - Marshmallow Fluff with a banana instead of Boston Cream Pie
    - Lite Cherry Pie Filling with Cool Whip instead of cherry pie and whipped cream
    - Pumpkin (with pumpkin pie spice) and Cool Whip instead of pumpkin pie
    - Edy's Fruit Bard or Jelly Belly Freezer Pops instead of ice cream
    - Dannon Lite & Fit Yogurt or Stonyfield Oikos Plain Greek Yogurt instead of ice cream
    - Seelect Pancake Syrup, Walden Farm Low Carb caramel dip for apple slices, bananas, oranges, pears, and other fruits

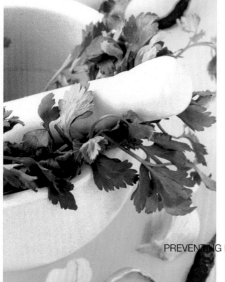

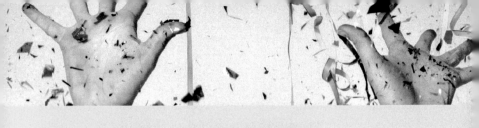

CHAPTER EIGHTEEN
RICER SUCCESS STORIES

I N 1940, THE LEGENDARY DR. WALTER KEMPNER INTRODUCED THE RICE DIET at the Duke University Medical Center. Since then, thousands and thousands of people have embraced the Rice Diet lifestyle to lose weight, reverse their medical conditions, and enjoy healthy, quality lives. We'd like you to meet some of these people, and be inspired by their own stories— stories of dreams, determination, challenges and success. Chances are, you'll see at least a part of your own story reflected in their words and experiences. This should tell you two things. First, you are not alone in your courageous battle to overcome obesity. And second, you too can author a story of triumph. You too can inspire others who will follow. You too can succeed. The following testimonials are from patients at the Rice Diet of Central Florida program.

ROBERT

By the age of 49, I'd already had a heart attack. I was on a lot of different medications, and I had high blood pressure, high cholesterol, GERD, heartburn, sleep apnea, early Type 2 diabetes and swelling of the feet. I was 100 pounds overweight, and I could barely walk up a flight of stairs to my condo without running out of breath.

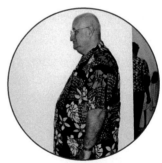

I started the Rice Diet and lost 12 pounds in the first week. I lost 31 pounds in the first month! My blood sugar went down from 146 to 102, I was able to walk two miles a day, and I no longer had GERD. Soon I was sleeping better and I was able to stop using my CPAP machine, which I used for sleep apnea. I was also able to stop taking these medications: spironolatone, Diovan®, potassium supplement, Tricor® and Zetia®.

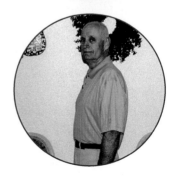

After nine months on the Rice Diet, I had gone from 275 pounds down to 173 pounds. My waist went from 48 inches down to 32 inches. I was walking six miles a day, doing work around the house that I could never do before, and even my arthritis improved.

Best of all, I feel ALIVE, with lots of energy and enthusiasm. I have now become the person I wanted to be all those years when I struggled with obesity and poor health.

EMMET

I was an athletic man for most of my life. By age 58 though, I was a mess. I weighed 290 pounds, had suffered a heart attack and had two stents in my coronary arteries. I had Type 2 diabetes and high cholesterol, I suffered from peripheral edema (leg swelling), and I needed a CPAP machine for sleep apnea. Then I started on the Rice Diet.

Nine months later, I had lost 85 pounds, down from 290 to 205. That's seven pounds less than I weighed at age 20 in the Marine Corps! My waist went from 51 inches down to 34, I'm off my diabetes and blood pressure medications, and I no longer need a CPAP machine to sleep. I enjoy daily exercise, and I play basketball with guys half my age. I'm happier than I have been years and years—this is the way to live.

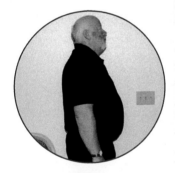

I've found the Rice Diet easy to follow and easy to do. What they say is true: stick with the program and it sticks with you. The Rice Diet has definitely been the right diet for me.

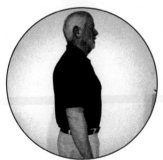

GWEN

I was 61 years old and depressed about being overweight. Most of my weight gain happened after age 40. I developed GERD, heartburn, arthritis and worsening irritable bowel syndrome. After nine months on the Rice Diet with my husband, I lost almost 50 pounds and seven inches from my waist. My spirits were improved, and my medical problems all improved and resolved for the most part. I was able to get off my heartburn medication completely. If I keep this up, I will be the healthiest I have been in years, and look and feel better than I have in a long time. My husband is so impressed with the new me! I feel so much younger. The struggle and persistence of sticking with the Rice Diet is absolutely worth it.

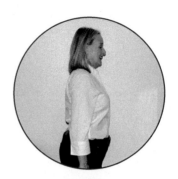
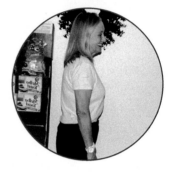

REBECA

I am a 42-year-old woman. I'm five feet tall and weighed 222 pounds before I began the Rice Diet. My obesity was due mostly to emotional overeating, and I had developed hypertension and Irritable Bowel Syndrome. Thanks to the Rice Diet, I was able to get control of my eating and emotions, and so far have lost 29 pounds in six weeks! My waist has gone from 42 inches to 37 inches and I got my IBS under control in a few weeks. My blood pressure gradually came down too—without medication! I feel great, I'm sleeping better and have more energy then I have in a decade. I was able to begin an exercise program and this is a lifestyle that I can live with for the rest of my life.

PEG

At age 62 I was 25 pounds overweight and had many medical issues: a history of a TIA (transient stroke), hypertension, high cholesterol, GERD, and arthritis. After 10 weeks on the Rice Diet, I lost 20 pounds (while eating out in restaurants many times a week!). I was able to eliminate two blood pressure medications, and my statin and arthritis medication. That saved me almost $400.00 per month in drug costs. I had more energy, no acid reflux symptoms, and I had more flexibility, strength, and ability to exercise. This is the best I have felt in my life.

BRUCE

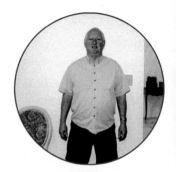

I am 63 years old, and I'm five-feet-seven inches tall. I weighed 217 pounds and had hypertension, severe GERD, high cholesterol, arthritis of the hips and fluid in my legs. On the Rice Diet I was able to lose 65 pounds, and now I am at my ideal body weight. For the first time in 20 years I can wash my feet in the shower and can go up many flights of stairs without being out of breath. I was able to get to normal blood pressure and get off two cholesterol medications, and still have normal blood work. I have now kept the weight off for more than nine months, and as long as I stick to the maintenance plan, I should be able to stay well for the rest of my life. This program changed my life!

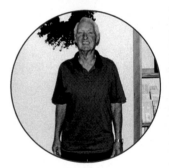

PAM

I am an 8th grade teacher who was basically crippled by arthritis. I am five-foot-four—and weighed 287 pounds (I once weighed 128 pounds). I had to take Tylenol®, Advil®, Nuprin® and Aleve® to get through the work day, because my knees hurt from carrying all that extra weight. After 8 months on the Rice Diet I lost 87 pounds, going from 286 to 199 pounds and dropping 11 inches from my waistline. Most important, I could work the entire day at school and not take any medication, and not have any knee pain. I had gone from being a binge eater to someone who could control my eating. The fact that I could buy all my food at the supermarket, and I could get it when I traveled or at home, made the Rice Diet a very easy diet for me, and now it is my lifestyle.

GRACE

I am 51 years old. I used to be slender at 5-foot-8 and 122 pounds. Then I suffered from a bout of depression after I got married, and gained 110 pounds. I had hypertension, asthma and arthritis. On the Rice Diet I was able to lose 45 pounds in five months. My arthritis improved to the point that I could stop taking meloxicam most of the time. When I was obese, I felt that I was a "big, powerful" person. As I lost weight however, I began to feel less powerful, and had to deal with this issue, which was a struggle. The support group at the Rice Diet has made this possible. Emotional support is a very important element of this program!

JIM

At age 63, I had 205 pounds on my five-foot-eight inch frame. I had arthritis in my knees, high blood pressure, elevated cholesterol, and was a heavy snorer. I needed to lose 55 pounds, and on the Rice Diet, I lost 40 pounds in nine months. I can walk without pain, and do not need any blood pressure medicine. I no longer snore and sleep much better. My cholesterol and triglycerides came back to normal. I've learned how to eat to live and not live to eat. I saw how the Rice Diet improved my health, and now my wife and I are sticking to this lifestyle!

BILL

I was 57 and had gained weight by working overtime and not having time to sit down and eat a healthy meal. I didn't exercise either. After years of this, I weighed 205 pounds (I'm five-feet-five inches tall). I had sleep apnea, elevated cholesterol, GERD, early coronary artery disease, and hypertension. Over the eight months I was on the Rice Diet, I was able to lose 62 pounds and ten-and-a-half inches from my waistline. There was complete resolution of the sleep apnea, I was able to get off my cholesterol medication, and never needed to begin blood pressure medication. I learned how to eat, and how to avoid all the pitfalls that caused me to get overweight and unhealthy in the first place. Through the group therapy I learned how to conduct my life and how to make my days full and happy, and eat healthily at the same time. I am happy to learn that this book is available for all those who can't join our group in Florida!

MARCIA

I am 67 and was suffering from arthritis, diabetes, elevated cholesterol, depression and irritable bowel syndrome. After one year on the Rice Diet program, I went from 195 pounds down to 145 pounds. My metabolism has always been so slow that weight loss was almost impossible. I have never exercised much but even so, I have lost 50 pounds, I have a normal blood pressure, and I'm off of my BP medication. I've also experienced a miraculous improvement in my irritable bowel syndrome since I started the Rice Diet, along with improvement in my self-esteem and feelings of well-being. I am better than I have been over the past 10-15 years, and I have more energy than I ever thought I would have. This experience has changed my life.

EVERETT

I am a 62 year old man who was a medical wreck. I had hypertension, Type 2 diabetes (but was on insulin), high cholesterol and sleep apnea. At 275 pounds, I was 100 pounds over my ideal body weight. Despite the fact that I was not a very good patient, I had amazing changes to my medical status. I only lost 18 pounds in six weeks, but in that time was able to stop my diuretics and high cholesterol medicine and cut my blood pressure medicine in half. I dropped my insulin from 120 to 25 units and my blood sugars dropped from 300 to 120 level. After one month I was able to decrease my Prilosec® from twice a day to once a day. I went from walking less than 1 block with shortness of breath to half a mile at a time without shortness of breath. Despite being a poor patient, I am incredibly impressed with the power of the diet to reverse my diseases. One can't say enough good things about the potential of the Rice Diet.

LINDA

I am 66 years old and looked and felt much older before I began on the rice diet program. I was 5 foot 3 inches tall and weighed over 160 pounds. My waist was 35 inches and I had a number of medical problems including high blood pressure, arthritis, high cholesterol and triglycerides and chronic reflux. It turns out I had early diabetes as well and fasting blood sugars in the 115 range. Shortly after starting the Rice Diet, I was no longer having heartburn. I had been taking TUMS and Rolaids relatively frequently but now no longer needed them. I was able to ultimately discontinue a blood pressure medicine and high cholesterol medication. I noticed that I was sleeping better, did not

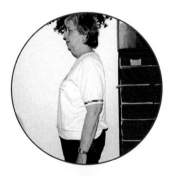

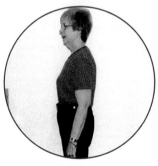

have the heartburn or indigestion and overall was feeling so much better. I was able to exercise and now I'm actually interested in exercising and do it on a regular basis. My waist went from 35 inches to 28 inches and I've lost 40 pounds over the last 7 months, and I am now at my ideal body weight. I am a new person with a new lifestyle and I owe it to the Rice Diet.

JANET

I am a 51-year-old woman who lost 20 pounds on the Rice Diet in three months. It was slow because I had to learn to overcome my emotional eating. With the group meetings and support of the professional staff, I am improving. My hypertension is now under control and I was able to stop taking my blood pressure medicine. My high cholesterol and triglycerides returned to normal. In fact, by changing my cooking habits and what food I bought for the house, my overweight husband lost 30 pounds, and he wasn't even on the program. He just ate the same foods that I did in larger amounts and began walking with me on a regular basis. Although he didn't have any medical problems to start with, he feels healthier and more energetic. This program is a blessing!

SANDI

I am a 53-year-old nurse who has battled weight for most of my life, since age 14. I am five-feet-five inches tall, and when I reached 214 pounds I knew I had to do something. At the time, I had high cholesterol, arthritis and hypertension; I had also had one knee replaced due to arthritis and was told I would need my other knee replaced as well. However, now that I have lost over 65 pounds on the Rice Diet, I don't think I'll need that second knee replacement! I have more energy than I did 10 years ago, and have stopped the cholesterol medication. My blood pressure is normal without medication and my arthritis is markedly improved. I am doing more exercise then I 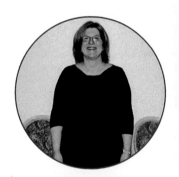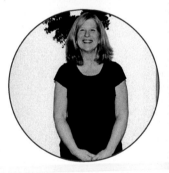 have ever been able to do. The Rice Diet is easy to follow and I enjoy the fact that it is a whole food diet that I can follow anywhere in the world. I look better and feel better, and my husband concurs!

TJ

I am a 35-year-old woman who is very overweight and wanted to have a child. I began the Rice Diet to lose weight before getting pregnant, since I was told I would be a high risk for gestational diabetes and pre-eclampsia. At first it was difficult, but soon, I had lost 28 pounds in two months and was feeling great. I had more energy, slept better (I had insomnia to start with), and was able to exercise for the first time in years. I was also able to control my hypertension without any medication. I learned to exercise, and how to say "no" to others who increased my stress levels. The fundamentals that I learned here have changed my life and my outlook.

CARL

I was 59 years old and realized that I was significantly overweight. I was very tall at 6 foot 6 inches and thought that I was able to carry a lot more weight than most people because of my height. I was 273 pounds and suffered from chronic gastroesophageal reflux since age 25. I had been having elevated blood sugar levels for some time but did not wish to start on any medication. I had high blood pressure and arthritis and found out that I had a fatty liver and elevated liver enzymes once I was put through some tests at the Rice Diet program. My blood sugar was in the 139 range but within 5 weeks on the diet I was able to get down to the normal range of 95. My diabetes was miraculously cured. Over the next 2 months, fatty changes in my liver resolved and my liver enzymes went back to normal. I was able to drop my waist from 48-1/2 inches to 39. I was able to discontinue Nexium for my chronic heartburn, and 2 blood pressure medications. Now after getting down from 273 to 218 pounds, I'm at my ideal body weight and feel terrific. I do not have high blood pressure, stopped snoring and feel great overall. I have learned to exercise on a regular basis and my eating habits are well ingrained. I am sure I will be able to continue this for the rest of my life.

For more success stories, including video testimonials, go to www.RiceDietCF.com

APPENDIX

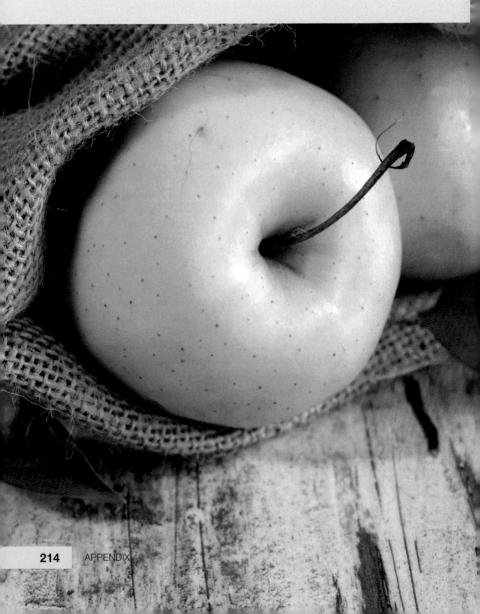

PRESCRIPTION FOR YOUR HEALTH

What is a prescription for good health? Do you have any thoughts about what you would write down on a prescription pad if you were the one making the recommendations? Would you consider writing down the following?

- Having a positive mental attitude to enable your healthy lifestyle.
- Engage in social interaction to stimulate your mind. Experience an interchange of thoughts, feelings, things in common, intellectual discussions and differences of opinion. To listen to someone when they are in need and to have someone listen to you when you are in need? To gain support, attention, respect, affection, love from another. To share experiences and life's challenges with others. Time alone to meditate, relax and do deep breathing.
- Volunteer time to a cause you believe in, to make a difference in another's life, or help those in need, at a school, homeless shelter, hospital, nursing home, etc.
- To participate and interact in stimulating games such as brain teasers, puzzles to keep your mind active and sharp. Challenge your mind.
- Maintain hobbies, interests, take classes for fun or to change or further your career.

Patient Name:_____
Address:_____Date:_____

Rx

Age: _____
Weight: _____
Goal Weight: _____

Height: ___ Waist: ___ Clothing Size: _____

Medications: _____
Blood Pressure: _____
Marital Status: _____
Employed/Retired: _____
Favorite Exercises: _____
Are you stressed: _____
Ways you deal with stress: _____

MD:_____
Signature:_____

- Consider having pets appropriate to your lifestyle, such as a fish, cat, dog or bird (depending on your daily schedule and needs of the pet) to enjoy companionship, caring for another, and walking your dog for exercise. Watching your fish swim could aid relaxation.
- Write a letter, email or call a friend. Stay connected with friends and relatives.
- Engage in physical activity on a daily basis; keep your body moving, no excuses. Go bike riding, walking, swimming, play tennis take dance lessons, etc.
- Make health a #1 priority over all else, for when ill, everything else will be difficult to do.
- Put things into perspective: choose health over the "taste" of food. Avoid foods high in salt, fat, and sugar. You won't crave eating more and will eventually develop new tastes and gain good health.
- Eat mindfully, practice portion control, monitor servings, keep hydrated, take a daily multiple vitamin, walk!
- Journal your eating, feelings, mistakes and how to correct it next time, stay positive, stay focused and do better the next meal. You matter. It doesn't matter what other people think about "your Rice Diet/healthy lifestyle," or if you don't eat enough, look too thin. Stay confident, stay strong. Stay the course, focus on being healthy, feeling good, looking good and living a healthy life to enjoy with your family, grandchildren, friends and doing all the things you enjoy doing in life.
- Make time and take time to take care of yourself.
- Maintain photos of yourself over time.

- Think before you eat. Are you really hungry? Delay for 15 minutes.
- Wear a pedometer: 10,000 steps equals 5 miles.
- Schedule your exercising and keep to it, enlist others to join you in walking/exercise class and don't cancel.
- Package foods in zip lock bags and containers for at home and on the go; always be prepared, plan ahead.
- Journal entries cause you to be true to yourself.
- Weigh yourself, don't let plateaus dampen spirits.
- Stay out of the kitchen at night, shut the lights, put a stop sign on the refrigerator door or a mirror inside.
- When enjoying time with family/friends, choose activities other than food.
- Avoid "sitting disease," move your body all the time.
- Once you've lost weight, reward yourself with non-food like a movie/book/belt)

POSITIVE THINKING AND POSITIVE AFFIRMATIONS

If you believe, you will achieve. Wouldn't it be wonderful if you could begin each day with a positive attitude? Well, it's not impossible. You can begin each day with a positive thought. Most beneficial in developing a positive outlook on life is employing positive affirmations.

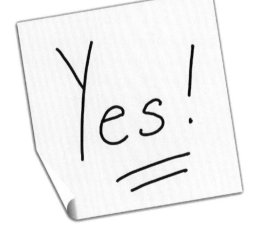

Positive affirmations are repeated positive thoughts that enable you to have a positive frame of mind and an inner peace. They are thoughts or statements about outcomes you wish to achieve. This will create a positive mind set, to better enable you to handle life's stresses, struggles, conflicts and challenges in a productive and healthy manner, and not cause you to resort to old ways, i.e. emotional eating. A positive mind set leads to positive outcomes.

Remember to make positive entries into your journals on a daily basis and when exercising, use positive affirmations as well.

Positive Affirmations to Employ:
- I deserve to be healthy
- I am feeling better and stronger each day
- I can eat healthy meals and determine I am full
- I can guard my regimen and avoid obstacles
- I can find things to do when tempted to eat
- I can enlist the support of others to strengthen me
- I can change
- I can give
- I can express my feelings
- I can find something positive about challenges
- I can strive to be an inspiration to others
- I can create a 'to do list' and get organized
- I am committed to living a healthy lifestyle
- I am open to new ideas
- I am committed to living a healthy lifestyle
- I am committed to losing weight to gain good health
- I am committed to adhering to the Rice Diet Program to achieve results
- I am committed to eating right and exercising right to get the right results

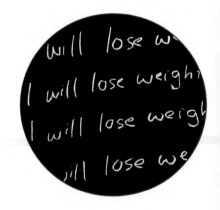

- I am committed to the commitment I made to myself and to value myself
- I am committed to guarding myself against obstacles from reaching my goal weight

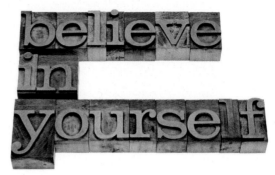

- I can celebrate my accomplishments in a non-food way, not resorting to my old ways
- I can exercise each day
- I can eat healthy meals
- I can guard my actions
- I can be true to myself
- I can hold myself accountable
- I can be proud of my daily willpower
- I can succeed
- I can receive
- I can assert myself
- I can take time for myself
- I can walk the walk
- I can find things to do when I'm bored
- I am committed to losing weight
- I am working toward my goals
- Life is getting better each day
- I am healthy and happy and energized

Create your own affirmations. Truly believe what you are affirming is attainable. Have a realistic plan to achieve your goal.

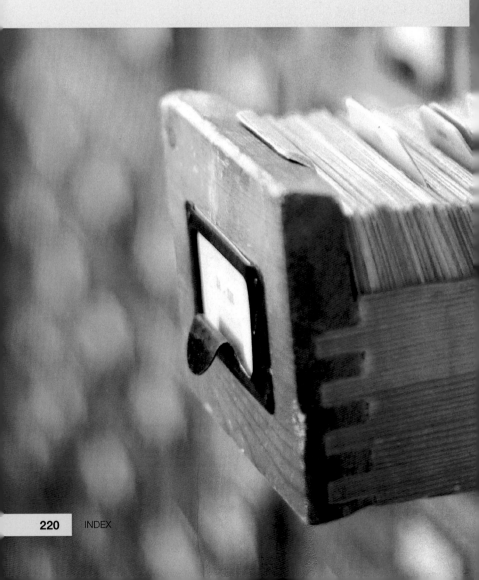

INDEX

REFERENCES

Sprung, D.J., Sprung, D.D. "Is Weight Reduction the Key Factor in Controlling GERD Symptoms in Obese Patients?" American Journal of Gastroenterology, Oct 2010, Vol. 105, No. S1, p. S27.

Sprung, D.J., Sprung, D.D. "Controlling Irritable Bowel Syndrome with the Rice Diet: A Pleasant Fringe Benefit." American Journal of Gastroenterology, Oct 2010, Vol. 105, No. S1, p. S502.

Kempner W. Treatment of kidney disease and hypertensive vascular disease with the Rice Diet. North Carolina Medical Journal 1944; 5: 125-33.

Kempner W. Treatment of kidney disease and hypertensive vascular disease with the Rice Diet, II. North Carolina Medical Journal 1944; 5: 272-74.

Kempner W. Treatment of cardiac failure with the Rice Diet. North Carolina Medical Journal 1947; 8: 128-31.

Kempner W. Treatment of hypertensive vascular disease with the Rice Diet. The American Journal of Medicine 1948; 4: 545-77. Reprinted in the Kempner Symposium, 1974.

Kempner W. Treatment of heart and kidney disease and of hypertensive and arteriosclerotic vascular disease with the Rice Diet. Annals of Internal Medicine 1949; 31: 821-56.

Kempner W., Lohmann-Peschel R., Schlayer C. Effect of Rice Diet on diabetes mellitus associated with vascular disease. Postgraduate Medicine 1958; 24: 359-71.

Kempner W. Effect of salt restriction on experimental nephrosis. Journal of the American Medical Association 1965; 191: 51.

Kempner W., Newborg B, Lohmann-Peschel R., Skyler JS. Treatment of massive obesity with rice/reduction program. Archives of Internal Medicine 1975; 135: 1575-84.

ABOUT THE RICE HOUSE

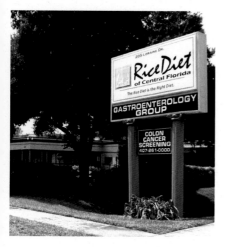

The Rice Diet of Central Florida conducts its program from within the walls of The Rice House, located in Altamonte Springs, Florida. Here, in a pleasant, cheerful environment, Dr. Sprung, Mrs. Sprung and their medical staff provide the education, supervision and motivation to help patients improve their health and transform their lives.

Each person who enters The Rice House is treated as an individual, receiving close, personal attention including regularly scheduled exams, weigh-ins, medical checks, educational lectures, group activities and more.

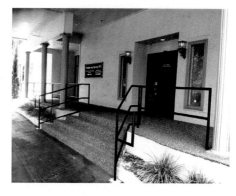

The Rice House is conveniently located near several hotels, walking areas, indoor exercise facilities, and an indoor air-conditioned mall for walking during inclement weather. Dr. and Mrs. Sprung have designed the Rice House to be a welcoming place of hope, positive activity and life transformation. So come visit, and leave a healthier, happier person. For life!

Call: (407) 261-0000
Click: www.RiceDietCf.com | info@ricedietcf.com
Visit: 205 Loraine Drive | Altamonte Springs, Florida 32701

ABOUT THE AUTHORS

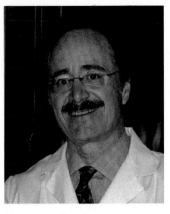

Douglas Jay Sprung, MD, FACG, FACP, is the medical director at the Rice Diet of Central Florida. He is a board-certified internist and gastroenterologist who trained at Duke University School of Medicine and studied with Dr. Walter Kempner, the originator of the Duke Rice Diet, then and during his subsequent residency training at Duke. His gastroenterology fellowship was done at the Lahey Clinic in Burlington, Massachusetts. In more than 25 years of private practice in Orlando, Florida, Dr. Sprung has observed first-hand the effectiveness of the Rice Diet in reversing obesity and related health problems. Dr. Sprung advocates the Rice Diet as a medically sound, practical and doable regimen to reverse obesity and achieve lifelong good health.

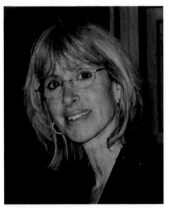

Denise Sprung, MSW, received her masters of social work at the University of North Carolina at Chapel Hill. She has an impressive background in education and healthcare, including training at the Duke University Comprehensive Cancer Center, the Durham VA Hospital and the University of North Carolina Memorial Hospital. Mrs. Sprung is the program director at the Rice Diet of Central Florida, assuming a wide range of responsibilities in patient education, nutrition, motivation and counseling. Mrs. Sprung's mission is to allow all patients to attain the skills needed to achieve their goals to lose weight, get healthy and be happy.

Both Dr. and Mrs. Sprung are "Ricers" as well, not only advocating, but living the "Ricer lifestyle."